JOHN EBNEZAR CBS | Handbooks in
Orthopedics and Fractures

SERIES

Orthopedic Problems of Different Ages

Orthopedic Problems of Public Health Importance

VOLUME IV

- Regional Conditions of the Spine
- Regional Conditions of the Upper Limb
- Regional Conditions of the Lower Limb
- Low Backache
- Miscellaneous Problems

John Ebnezar

- Holder of the **Guinness Book of World Records** for the most number of books written by an individual in a single year.
- Listed in the **India Book of Records** for the most number of books written by an individual.
- Recipient of the highest civilian awards of Karnataka, the **Rajyotsava Award 2010** and the **Kempegowda Award 2011**.
- Recipient of the **Best Citizen of India Award** by the International Publishing house.
- Former Vice-President, the Indian Orthopaedic Association
- President, Neuro-Spinal Surgeons Association of India (Karnataka)
- CEO, Parimala Health Care Services, A ISO 9001:2008 Hospital, Bilekahalli, Bannerghatta Road, Bangalore
- Ebnezar Orthopedic Center, Bilekahalli, Bannerghatta Road, Bangalore
- Dr John's Orthopedic Clinic, near Reliance Mart, Arakere, BG Road, Bangalore
- Chairman, the Physically Handicapped and Paraplegic Charitable Trust of Karnataka®
- Founder President, Geriatric Orthopedic Society
- Founder President, Orthopedic Authors Association and All India Medical Authors Association
- Chairman, Karnataka Orthopedic Academy®
- President, Bangalore Holistic Academy
- Chairman, Rakesh Cultural Academy
- President, Vaidya Kala Ranga, Bangalore
- Secretary, SK Educational Society®
- Former Senior Specialist, Victoria Hospital, Bangalore Medical College, Bangalore
- Former Assistant Professor in Orthopedics, Devaraj Urs Medical College, Kolar, Karnataka
- Postgraduate teacher, Bangalore Baptist Hospital, Airport Road, Bangalore

John Ebnezar CBS | Handbooks in Orthopedics and Fractures

SERIES

Orthopedic Problems of Different Ages

Orthopedic Problems of Public Health Importance

Volume IV

- Regional Conditions of the Spine
- Regional Conditions of the Upper Limb
- Regional Conditions of the Lower Limb
- Low Backache • Miscellaneous Problems

John Ebnezar

MBBS, D'Ortho, DNB (Ortho), MNAMS (Ortho), PhD (Yoga)
Sports Medicine (Australia), INOR Fellow (UK), DAc, DMT

Consulting Orthopedic and Spine Surgeon
Holistic Orthopedic Expert, and Sports Specialist
Bangalore

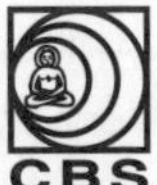

CBS Publishers & Distributors Pvt Ltd

New Delhi • Bengaluru • Pune • Kochi • Chennai

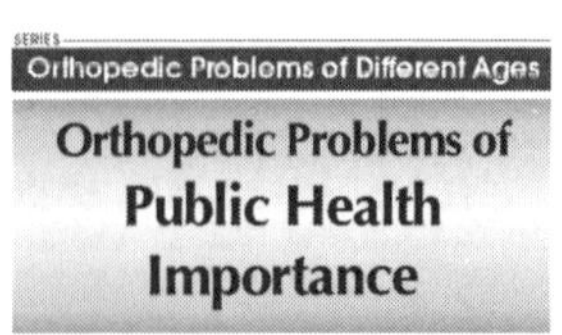

VOLUME IV

ISBN: 978-81-239-2165-5

First Edition: 2012

Published by Satish Kumar Jain and produced by Vinod K. Jain for
CBS Publishers & Distributors Pvt Ltd
4819/XI Prahlad Street, 24 Ansari Road, Daryaganj
New Delhi 110 002, India.
Website: www.cbspd.com
Ph: 23289259, 23266861, 23266867
e-mail: delhi@cbspd.com
Fax: 011-23243014
cbspubs@airtelmail.in.

Branches

- Bengaluru: Seema House 2975, 17th Cross, K.R. Road, Banasankari 2nd Stage, Bengaluru 560 070, Karnataka
  Ph: +91-80-26771678/79 Fax: +91-80-26771680 e-mail: bangalore@cbspd.com
- Pune: Bhuruk Prestige, Sr. No. 52/12/2+1+3/2 Narhe, Haveli (Near Katraj-Dehu Road Bypass), Pune 411 051, Maharashtra
  Ph: 020-64704058, 64704059, 32392277 Fax: +91-020-24300160 e-mail: pune@cbspd.com
- Kochi: 36/14 Kalluvilakam, Lissie Hospital Road, Kochi 682 018, Kerala
  Ph: +91-484-4059061-65 Fax: +91-484-4059065 e-mail: cochin@cbspd.com
- Chennai: 20, West Park Road, Shenoy Nagar, Chennai 600 030, Tamil Nadu
  Ph: +91-44-26260666, 26208620 Fax: +91-44-45530020 email: chennai@cbspd.com

Printed at Magic International, Greater Noida (UP)

to

---

my mother
(late) Sampath Kumari
who taught me that life is more than self and
there is more joy in giving and sharing than taking

my wife
Dr Parimala

my lovely children
Rakesh and Priyanka
who are an epitome of love, sacrifice, encouragement
and inspiration

all my teachers
who made me what I am today

all my students
past and present

and

all my patients

Dr John Ebnezar

is a legendary name as a prolific orthopedic writer. No other orthopedic surgeon in the world has come anywhere close to him in the number of books he has written in his field. He is the first orthopedic surgeon in the world to be listed in the **Guinness Book of World Records** for the most number of books written by an individual in a single year. For the same feat his name has been listed in the **India Book of Records.** This book, like all his previous books, carries his flavor of simple and lucid writing, excellent language, beautiful illustrations and excellent presentation of the topics. This book is a part of the 100^{+} book series he has brought out in a single calendar year of 2012 on a wide array of orthopedic problems of public health importance. No other individual in the world has brought out these many books in one year and this is a world record attempt. With these books he aims to educate the reader and the public about these common orthopedic problems.

All his books have been accepted very well and he has a great fan following all over the world. He has been bestowed with as many as 32 international, national and state awards including Karnataka state's highest civilian award the **Rajyotsava Award 2010** and the **Kempegowda Award 2011,** apart from the **Best Citizen of India Award** given by the International Publishing House. He is the pioneer in holistic orthopedics and is credited for discovering a new method of treatment for the common orthopedic problems and has done PhD in arthritis from the world famous S-VYASA University, Bangalore. He is currently president of the Neuro-Spinal Surgeons Association of India (Karnataka), the former Vice-President of the Indian Orthopedic Association, and is the founder president of various orthopedic bodies.

Preface

This book is a part of the 100+ book series

John Ebnezar CBS Handbooks in Orthopedics and Fractures

which deals with the orthopedic problems of public health importance. The purpose of these books is to educate and create awareness among the readers about various problems associated with orthopedics. Through this way the readers get to know all about various orthopedic problems directly from a specialist. This will help a reader immensely in getting the right knowledge as most of them depend on the internet and magazines which distort and misrepresent various pieces of information concerning health topics, leaving the readers confused and worse still improperly educated. This may harm more than helping them find solutions to their problems. The purpose of these books, therefore, is to educate the readers right in their quest for knowledge on the common health and associated problems.

The 100+ book series has been brought out in a single calendar year.

This is a unique book, first of its kind that deals with the various common orthopedic problems of public health importance encountered in the society. This book gives an insight into various orthopedic problems peculiar to the society, their cause, presentation, investigations, treatment, complications and their impact on the individual health and the society in general. This is the first ever book which exclusively deals with all the common orthopedic problems of public health importance. Many of my patients were asking for a book on this topic so that they could understand all about the common public health orthopedic problems that are exclusively or more commonly seen in the society and the role they need to play in their prevention and treatment.

Highlights of this book

- Simple and lucid language
- Good illustrations

- Good Clinical photograph wherever necessary
- Relevant X-rays
- Short summaries
- Anecdotes
- Suggestions for self-help techniques

This book has ubiquitous utility and usage and can be useful to the orthopedic surgeons, postgraduate students in orthopedics, undergraduate medical students, doctors from all disciplines of medicine, physiotherapists, therapists practising alternative systems of medicine, rehabilitation specialists, and most importantly the common people. It is particularly useful to those unsung heroes who work in remote areas with minimum infrastructure. They can use this book as a ready-reckoner. Seldom will you find a book that covers such a wide spectrum of readers.

Knowing all about various orthopedic problems of public health importance creates an awareness and helps one to prevent most of these problems from happening at the first place.

Please remember that this book is meant to educate and not substitute the role of a doctor. I advise you to see your orthopedic surgeons if you are suffering from any of the cmmon orthopedic problems and use this book to update your knowledge about the condition and practice simple self-help techniques apart from adhering to the do's and don'ts for each condition.

Constructive criticism and useful suggestions are invited to make the book more effective in its forthcoming editions.

John Ebnezar

Acknowledgments

This volume is a part of the 100+ book series brought out in a single calendar year. This was a huge and mammoth task attempted first time ever by an author and a publisher in the world. Such an herculean effort could not have been possible without the active involvement of those concerned in CBS Publishers & Distributors. I thank Mr Satish K Jain, Managing Director of CBS P&D, for agreeing to be a part of this world-record feat in bringing out this book in the Series. My special thanks to Mr YN Arjuna who showed special interest in this work and channelized his entire energy into this improbable feat. My special thanks to Mrs Ritu Chawla and her entire dedicated team who have toiled day and night to make this dream a reality. I thank members of the entire editorial–production team of CBS P&D who have worked hard behind the scenes to bring out this book.

My special thanks to Dr Yogitha for actively helping me in the compilation of all the books. I also thank all the staff members of my hospital who have helped me at various levels during the making of this book.

John Ebnezar

Contents

John Ebnezar **CBS** Handbooks in

Orthopedics and Fractures

TITLES IN THE SERIES

I Orthopedic Trauma

General Fractures

1 General Principles of Fractures and Dislocations
2 Fracture Treatment Methods
3 Fractures and their Complications
4 Atypical Fractures

Injuries of Upper Limb

5 Injuries of Shoulder
6 Injuries of Arm
7 Injuries of Elbow
8 Injuries of Forearm
9 Injuries of Wrist and Hand
10 Injuries of Distal Forearm and Wrist
11 Injuries of Hand
12 Injuries of Upper Limb

Injuries of Lower Limb

13 Injuries of Hip
14 Injuries of Femur
15 Injuries of Knee
16 Injuries of Knee and Leg
17 Injuries of Ankle and Leg
18 Injuries of Foot and Ankle
19 Injuries of Lower Limb

Injuries of Axial Skeleton

20 Injuries of Pelvis and Hip
21 Injuries of Spine
22 Injuries of Pelvis and Spine

23 Sports Injuries Volume I
24 Sports Injuries Volume II
25 Soft Tissue Problems in Orthopedics
26 Geriatric Trauma
27 Pediatric Trauma

II Orthopedic Disease

28 Congenital Orthopedic Problems
29 Developmental Orthopedic Problems

VI Practical Examination

VII Orthopedic Problems of Different Ages

VIII Common Orthopedic Problems

IX Yoga Therapy in Common Orthopedic Problems

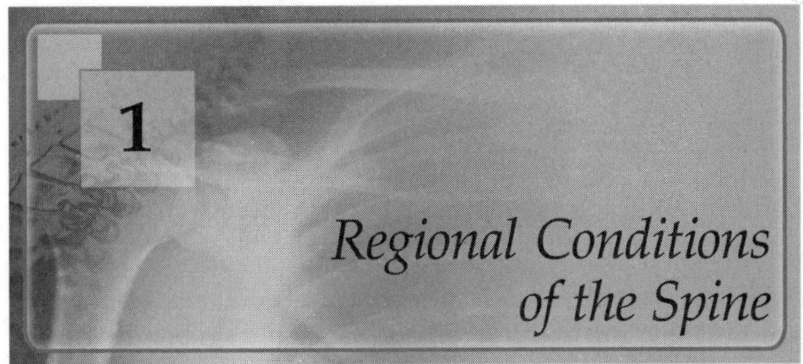

1 Regional Conditions of the Spine

SCOLIOSIS

Introduction

By definition, scoliosis is the lateral curvature of the spine in the upright position in the coronal plane. The lateral curvature is usually accompanied by some rotational deformity. Only man boasts of an erect posture. Nature has designed four physiological curves in the so-called erect spine, cervical and lumbar lordosis, dorsal curve in the thoracic spine and the sacral region. Thus, when the spine develops a lateral curve, it is abnormal. It throws the well-adjusted spinal mechanism out of gear and poses the following problems:

- A cosmetically unacceptable deformity.
- Deranges the load and force transmission mechanism through the spine.
- Jeopardizes the functions of vital organs like lungs, heart by overcrowding the ribs.
- Managing it is cumbersome and unrewarding experience most of the times.

Thus, a scoliotic curve makes the spine 'crooked' and a 'crooked spine is a wicked spine', if one considers the above problems it poses.

Varieties

Structural scoliosis: In structural scoliosis, the curves are fixed and nonflexible and fail to correct with side bending. Lateral

Mystifying facts

Do you know the difference between scoliosis and spinal asymmetry?
- Lateral curve $< 10^\circ$ — is spinal asymmetry.
- Lateral curve $> 10^\circ$ — is scoliosis.

bending of spine is asymmetric or involved vertebrae are fixed in a rotated position or both.

Nonstructural scoliosis: In nonstructural scoliosis, the curves are flexible and readily correctible with side bending. It is frequently seen as a compensatory mechanism to a leg length discrepancy, fixed flexion deformity of the hip (compensatory scoliosis), local inflammation or irritation due to acute lumbar disk disease and prolapsed disk (sciatic scoliosis) or due to poor postural habits (postural scoliosis).

Note:
- Postural scoliosis is the most common variety of nonstructural scoliosis.
- Idiopathic scoliosis is the most common variety of structural scoliosis.

Structural scoliosis may occur from a variety of causes. Idiopathic scoliosis accounts for 90 percent of all scoliosis and appears to represent a hereditary disorder, but the exact mechanism of its production is unknown. Broadly speaking, there are two types of scoliosis:
- Idiopathic (unknown cause).
- Known cause. The important among these are:
  - *Congenital scoliosis:* This is due to defect in segmentation, which is usually due to a lateral bar or due to a defect in the formation, including hemivertebrae or double hemivertebrae. These curves usually progress very fast and require surgical fusion on both the convex and concave sides of the curve.
  - *Paralytic scoliosis:* This is due to muscle imbalance on either side of the trunk, the most common cause being

anterior poliomyelitis. Cerebral palsies, muscular dystrophies, etc. are the other common causes.

Some of the other causes are mentioned at the end of the chapter.

Idiopathic scoliosis (unknown cause): This is the most common (75–90%) and three varieties are recognized—infantile, juvenile and adolescent. Though the exact cause is not known, role of genetics is hotly debated. Overall incidence is 1–4 people/thousand.

Clinical Features

Though idiopathic scoliosis can occur at any age, it usually appears clinically between 10 and 13 years. It is more common in females (10%). The disease is usually asymptomatic and is usually accidentally discovered. The diagnosis is usually made on routine physical examination (Figs 1.1A and B).

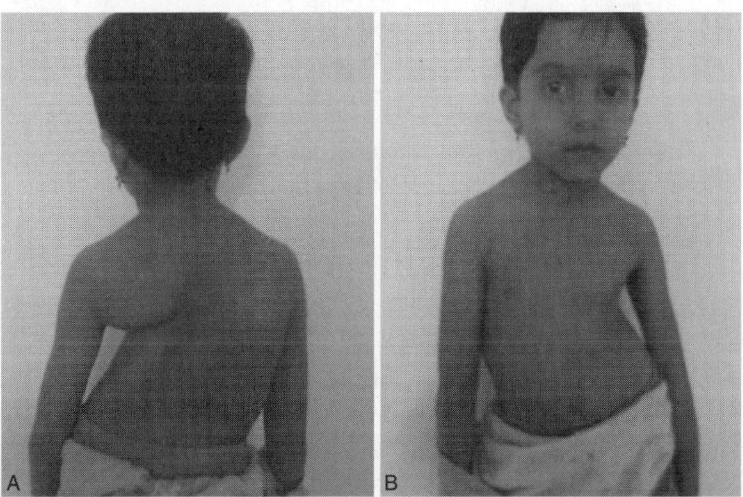

Figs 1.1A and B: (A) Scoliosis from back, (B) Scoliosis viewed from front (clinical photo)

Method of examination: For the examination, the patient should be undressed to the waist or wear a bathing suit and a routine should be followed. The shoulders and iliac crest are inspected to determine whether they are at the same level. The scapulae, ribcage and flanks are then observed for symmetry. The spinous processes are palpated to determine their alignment. Rib hump or abnormal paraspinal muscular prominence indicates spinal rotation. Rib hump leads to asymmetry of the trunk and is called angle trunk rotation (ATR). It is measured by using a scoliometer. The patient is then made to bend forward to see for the disappearance of the curve (Adam's test).

Scoliotic Facts

Structural curve: This is a laterally curved spine that lacks normal flexibility.
Primary care: This is the earliest curve to appear.
Compensatory curve or secondary curve: This is the curve, which develops above or below the primary curve in an effort to balance the spine.
Major curve: This is the largest structural curve.
Minor curve: This is the smallest curve.
Apical vertebra: This is the most deviated vertebra from the vertical axis of the patient.
End vertebrae

- The uppermost vertebra whose superior surface tilts maximally towards the concavity of the curve.
- The lowermost vertebra whose inferior surface tilts maximally towards the concavity of the curve.

Quick facts

Curve patterns in idiopathic scoliosis (Figs 1.2A to D)

Curve	*Apical vertebra*
Cervical	C_1–C_6
Cervicodorsal	C_7–T_1
Thoracic	T_2–T_{11}
Thoracolumbar	T_{12}–L_1
Lumbar	L_2–L_4
Lumbosacral	L_5–S_1

How to describe a scoliotic curve?

Remember the mnemonic PLEAD

- P—Pattern (primary, secondary, etc.)
- L—Location (thoracic, thoracolumbar lumbar)
- E—Etiology (idiopathic, congenital, paralytic, etc.)
- A—Apex (thoracic lumbar)
- D—Direction (right, left)

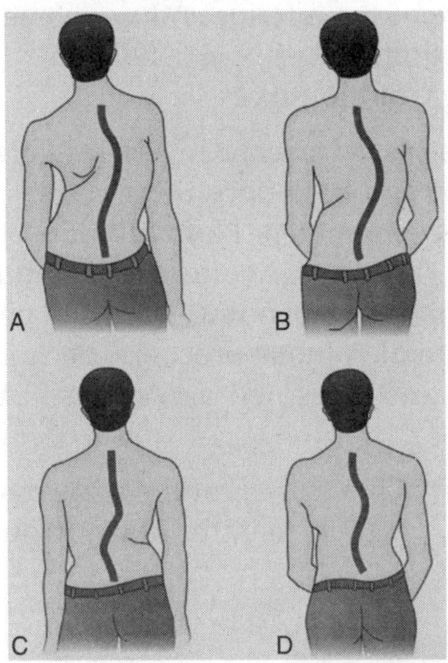

Figs 1.2A to D: (A) Various types of scoliosis: (A) Thoracic, (B) Thoracolumbar, (C) Double curve thoracic and lumbar, (D) Lumbosacral

Radiology

Radiographic evaluation of the spine is the only available method to determine the severity of the curve. It is repeated at intervals to determine the progression of the curve.

In radiography of the spine, the following views are taken. *PA view* of the spine (Fig. 1.3), standard lateral radiography of the spine, right and left bending films of spine and the Stagnara derotation view, which is an oblique view of the spine. The radiological parameters of importance are:

Cobb's method to measure severity of the curve: The upper and lower vertebrae are identified (Fig. 1.4). The upper end vertebra is the highest one whose superior border converges towards the concavity of the curve and the lower end vertebra is the one whose inferior border converges towards the concavity. Intersecting perpendicular line from the superior surface of the superior end vertebrae and from the inferior surface of the inferior end vertebrae is drawn. The angle of deviation of these perpendiculars from a straight line is the 'angle of the curve'.

Nash and Moe's method to measure vertebral rotation: In the PA view (Figs 1.5A and B) the positions of the spinous process and the pedicles are noted. Normally, the spinous process lies in the center. The apical vertebrae are graded for rotation on a scale from 0–4, depending upon the pedicle shadows and the position of spinous process. The spinous processes are identified and classified according to the amount of rotation.

Reisser's sign: This is a classification of the ossification of the iliac epiphysis, which usually starts from the anterior

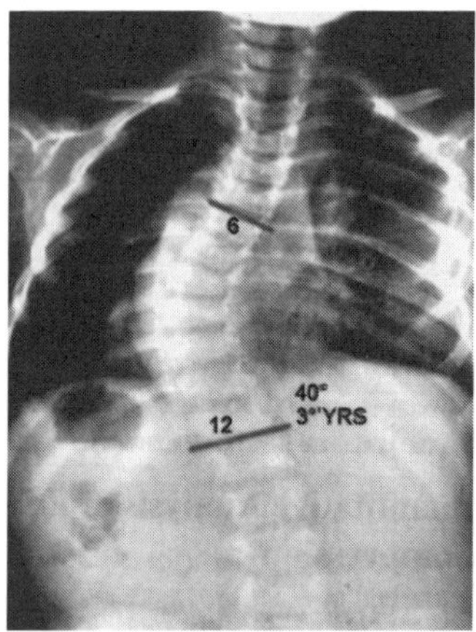

Fig. 1.3: Radiograph showing a paralytic scoliosis

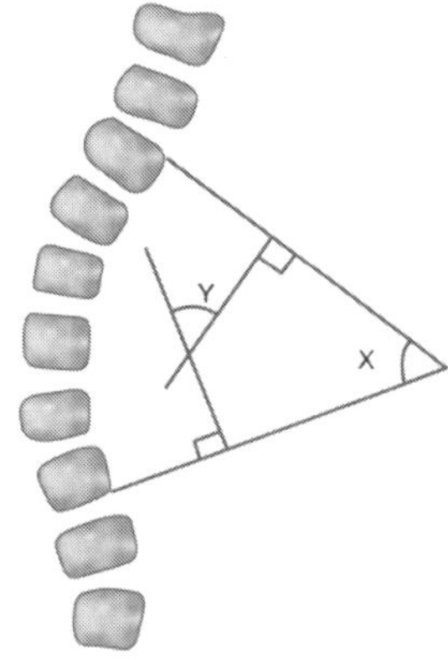

Fig. 1.4: Cobb's methods of measuring severity of a curve (Y = angle)

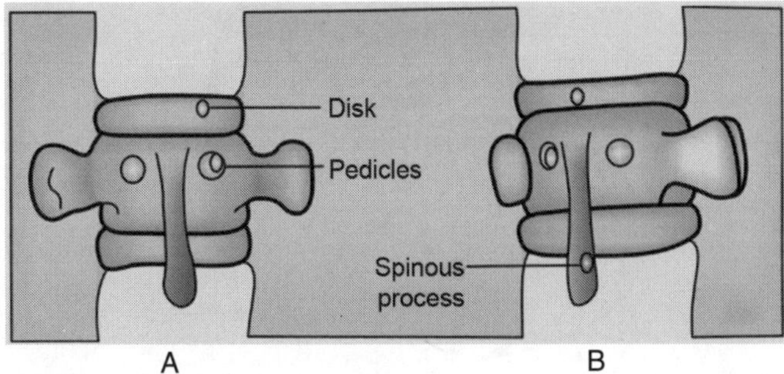

Figs 1.5A and B: (A) Normal PA view of the spine showing the normal positions of the pedicles and spinous processes, (B) The pedicles and spinous processes shadows are altered and indicate vertebral rotation in scoliosis

superior iliac spine and progresses posteriorly towards the posterior iliac spine. Reisser's stage 4 corresponds with cessation of spine growth and stage 5 correlates with cessation of height increase. *The importance of this sign is the completion of growth can be radiologically assessed which indicates no possibility of the curve progression.*

Reisser's classification

It uses ossification of iliac apophysis to grade the remaining skeletal growth. The ossification progresses from lateral to medial:

Type I — Ossification of lateral 25 percent
Type II — Ossification of lateral 50 percent
Type III — Ossification of lateral 75 percent
Type IV — Ossification of lateral 100 percent
Type V — Fusion of ilium

Rib angle of Mehta: The rib vertebral angle is constructed by the intersection of a line perpendicular to the apical vertebral end plate with a line drawn from the midneck to the midhead of the corresponding rib. The rib vertebral angle difference (RVAD) is the difference between rib vertebral angle of the convex and concave side of the apical vertebra. If the initial RVAD is less than 20°, progression is unlikely; and if initial RVAD is more than 20°, the curves tend to progress (Fig. 1.6).

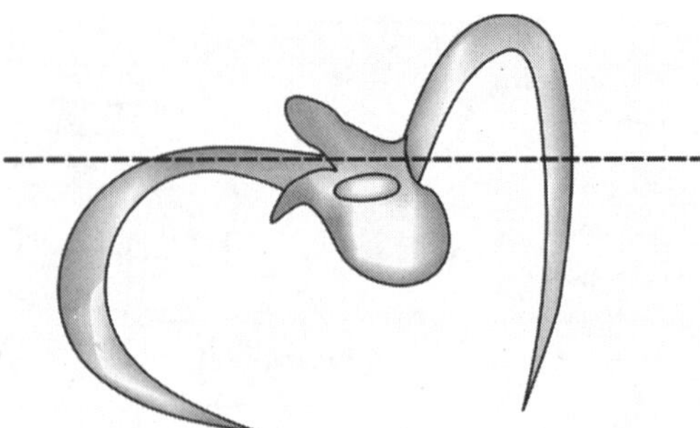

Fig. 1.6: Rib distortion due to vertebral rotation

Original structural curves are distinguished from secondary curves by the following criteria

- Vertebrae in structural scoliosis are displaced to the convexity of the curve; but in secondary curve, they are displaced to the concavity of the secondary curve.
- When there are three curves, *middle* one is structural.
- When there are four curves, *two middle* ones are structural.
- The greater curve or the one towards which the *trunk is shifted is the structural curve.*
- The curve that is flexible and corrective is the non-structural curve.

Compensation

If head is to be balanced above the pelvis when the patient is erect, it is done so by any curve or curves that develops in the opposite direction. *The formation of curves in the opposite direction is called compensation.* The angle of the secondary curves should be equal to that of the primary curve. If it exceeds, it is called overcompensation.

Treatment

The most important aspect in the treatment of scoliosis is early detection of the curve. A curve that is obvious in standing position has already approached 30–40°. *Detecting a curve before it reaches 20° is of utmost importance because curves over 20° tend to progress.* Frequent re-examinations are essential.

The treatment depends on the age of the patient and the severity of the curve.

Nonsurgical treatment: Observation is the primary treatment of all curves and more so for curves less than 20 degrees. *At present, radiography is the only definite documentation of curve size and progression.*

Generally accepted guidelines for observation

- Curves of less than 20° in skeletally immature persons are examined every 6 months.
- Curves less than 20° in skeletally mature persons require no further evaluation.
- Curves more than 20° in skeletally immature patients should be examined every 3–4 months. Orthotic treatment for curves more than 25°.
- Curves more than 30–40° in skeletally mature persons do not require treatment. However, they are examined radiographically for progression every 2–3 years.

Orthotic treatment: This is effective in skeletally immature persons (Figs 1.7A and B). For mild or moderate curves, 1Milwaukee brace, Boston brace, Reisser's turn buckle cast, localizer cast, etc. are used and the 20° level is considered still for bracing.

Remember

The 'Orthotic' leaders: Mnemonic BMC

B—Boston braces (TLSO)
M—Milwaukee brace
C—Carleston brace
Most effective among these is the Boston brace.

Do you know?

Complications of bracing?

- Most common: Discomfort and rejection due to poor appearance.
- Skin breakdown
- Excessive sweating
- Allergic skin reaction
- Increased gastric pressure and gastroesophageal reflex
- Spontaneous sternum fracture.

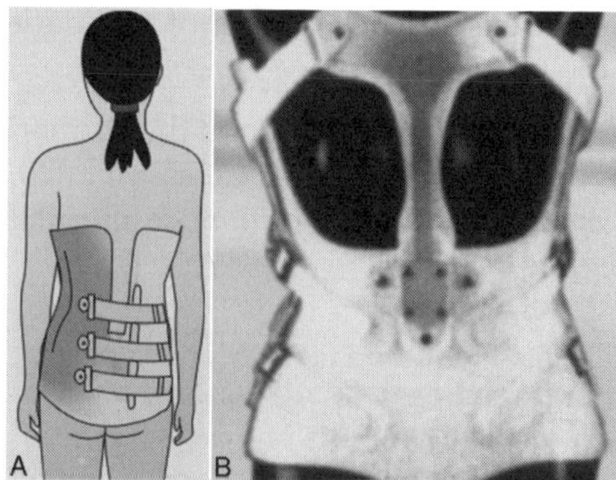

Figs 1.7A and B: (A) Orthotic treatment of structural scoliosis with Boston brace, (B) Brace for scoliosis

Other nonoperative measures: Exercises, traction and electrical stimulation have been unsuccessfully tried in adolescent variety.

Traction

Traction helps to stretch the contracted structures prior to surgery. Methods of traction could be either non-skeletal or skeletal. Skeletal traction is provided by halopelvic or halofemoral traction (Fig. 1.7C).

Mystifying facts: About braces

- Do you know what curves respond best to bracing?
  - Curves < 40°
  - Less severe lumbar hyperlordosis
  - Curves with thoracic lordosis
  - Hyperkyphosis
  - Risser's curve is 0
- How much is the efficacy of bracing?
  It is about 74 to 81 percent when worn for 23 hours/day until skeletal maturity.
- How do braces act?
  By derotating the spine using the rib or transverse process as the lever
- What are the corrective forces?
  The primary corrective forces are the 'lateral forces' in the braces.

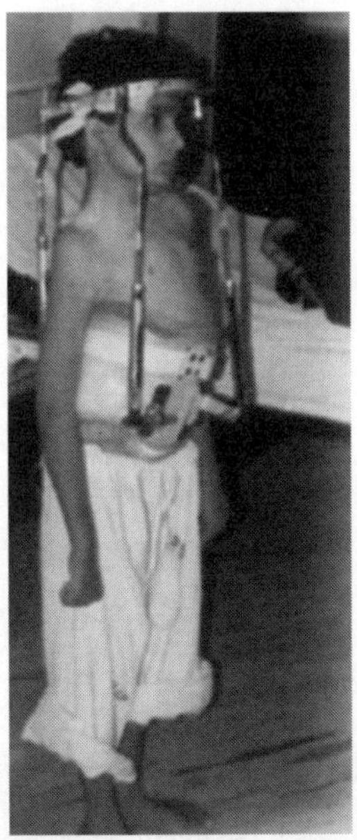

Fig. 1.7C: Halopelvic distraction apparatus used for skeletal traction in correction of structural scoliotic curves

Surgical treatment: This is indicated for high degree thoracic curve, which is inflexible and is associated with secondary changes in the ribs. Casts are not effective in thoracic spine. Spinal surgery is also indicated when the curve is over 60° and aims at obtaining fusion at the spine (*see box*) (Fig. 1.8).

Do you know in scoliosis?

- The proper indications for surgery?
  - Curves > 50° in the mature patients
  - Curves > 10° with marked rotations
  - Double major curves > 30°
- The most common form of surgical intervention in idiopathic scoliosis.

  Well, it is the segmental instrumentation with multiback system (CD).

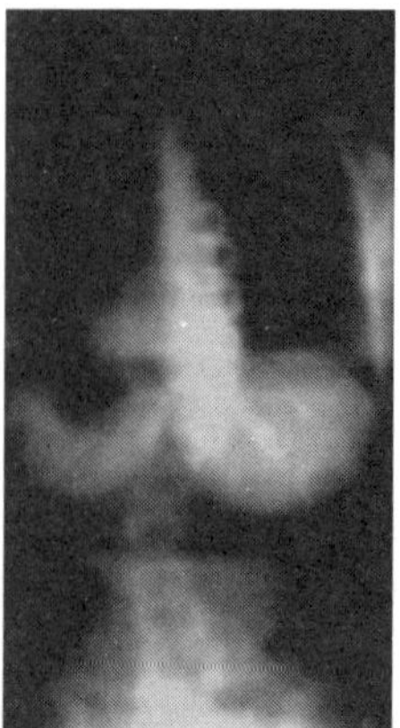

Fig. 1.8: Radiograph showing scoliosis surgical correction by segmental instrumentation

Methods of scoliosis treatment	
Distraction techniques	*Surgical fusion (Indications)*
• Rarely used • Spinal instrumentation and spinal cord monitoring have been developed **Methods** 1. Halopelvic distraction 2. Halofemoral distraction	• Too late for Milwaukee brace, > 15 years, > 50° curves • Failure to respond to Milwaukee brace • Curves > 60° • Pain in adults • Paralytic and congenital scoliosis (Fig. 1.3)

Methods		
Indications	*Anterior fusion*	*Posterior fusion*
• Kyphosis • Rigid scoliosis > 100° • Salvage procedure following failed spinal surgery. • Unstable spine due to laminectomy		• Harrington's instrumentation • Dwyer's instrumentation • Zielke's instrumentation • Hartshill rings, etc. • Segmental (Cotrel Duboucet system)

Quick facts

- Scoliosis is lateral curvature of the spine.
- Idiopathic variety accounts for 90 percent of the cases.
- Female preponderance.
- X-ray is the only definite documentation of curve size and progression.
- The most important aspect of treatment is early detection.
- Curves < 20° need observation.
- Curves > 20° require treatment.
- Curves between 20 and 40° can be treated by Milwaukee brace, which has to be worn 23 hours per day for a period of at least two years.
- Curves > 40° need surgical correction and fusion.

Facts about curve progression

- Curves < 20° will improve spontaneously in over 50 percent of cases.
- No accurate method to predict the outcome of curve.
- Twenty percent curves < 30° will progress.
- Progression is more common in young children.
- Bigger the curve at detection, higher is the chance of curve progression.
- Curve in females and double curves are more likely to progress.

Scoliosis of known cause: Congenital/paralytic.

Neuromuscular scoliosis

- *Neuropathic causes:* Spinal cord injury, poliomyelitis, progressive neurological disorders, syringomyelia, myelomeningocele and cerebral palsy are some of the neuropathic causes.
- *Muscular:* AMC and muscular dystrophy are some of the important muscular causes.
- *Neurofibromatosis.*
- *Miscellaneous:* Multiple epiphyseal dysplasias, osteogenesis imperfecta, etc.

Interesting facts

Remember 3 'O's in the treatment of idiopathic scoliosis:

- Observation for curves < 20°
- Orthosis for curves for > 20°–50°
- Operations for curves > 50°.

In a nutshell

Treatment options in scoliosis

Congenital	—	Surgery/bracing
Paralytic	—	Wheelchair seating systems
	—	Bracing, surgery
Idiopathic	—	3 'O's mentioned earlier
Marked rotation	—	Bracing
Degenerative		
< 60 years	—	Postural correction, exercises, corset, etc.
> 60 years	—	Surgery

Alternative therapies: Exercises, electric stimulation, biofeedback, tractions, manipulations, etc.

Unfavorable prognostic factors in scoliosis

- Congenital/juvenile/paralytic
- > 20–40° curve
- Thoracic curve
- 2–4 degree of rotation
- Risser's sign of immature
- Female
- Premenarchial
- Presence of osteoporosis
- Rapid increase in curve size
- Single short curve
- Previous discectomy, laminectomy, etc.

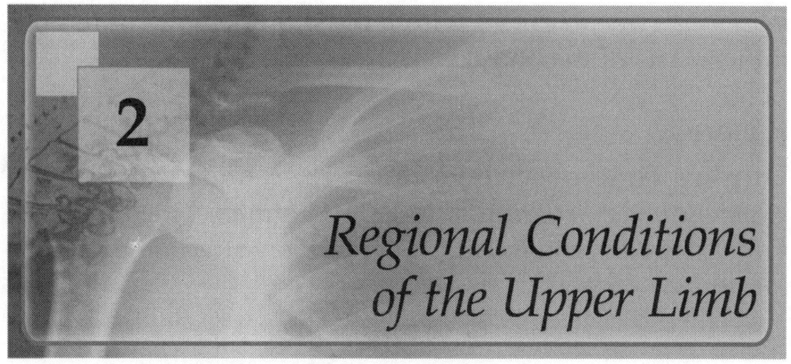

2 Regional Conditions of the Upper Limb

FROZEN SHOULDER

(Syn: Periarthritis, Adhesive Capsulitis)

Introduction

Paradoxically shoulder joint privileged as the most mobile joint in the body has its nemesis because of this very advantage. Its mobility makes it very vulnerable to problems, which ultimately "freezes" its movements. Unable to come to terms with the paucity of liberal movements hitherto enjoyed, the hapless patient resigns himself or herself to suffer the agony in silence!

It is defined as a clinical syndrome characterized by *painful restriction* (Figs 2.1A and B) *of both active and passive shoulder*

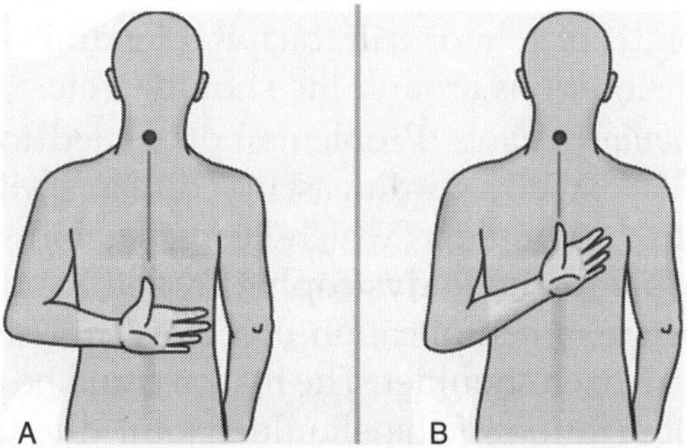

Figs 2.1A and B: Test to detect frozen shoulder (note the distance between the thumbs): (A) Frozen shoulder, (B) Normal

movements due to causes within the shoulder joint or remote (other parts of the body).

History

Dupley first described it in 1872 and called it as *humeroscapular periarthritis.* In 1934, **Codman** coined the term *Frozen shoulder*, and in 1945, **Neviaser** gave the name *adhesive capsulitis*.

Epidemiology of Frozen Shoulder

- Incidence in general population is 2 percent.
- Incidence in diabetics is 10–35 percent.
- More common in females than males.
- Mean age is 40–60 years.
- Bilateral 12 percent.

Causes

The causes for frozen shoulder could be:

- ***Primary:*** Here the exact cause is not known and it could be idiopathic.
- ***Secondary:*** According to **Lumberg,** the secondary causes could be:
  - *Shoulder causes:* Problems directly related to shoulder joint which can give rise to frozen shoulder are tendonitis of rotator cuff, bicipital tendinitis, fractures and dislocations around the shoulder, etc.
  - *Nonshoulder causes:* Problems not related to shoulder joint like diabetes, cardiovascular diseases with referred pain to the shoulder, which keeps the joint immobile, reflex sympathetic dystrophy, frozen hand shoulder syndrome, a complication of Colles' fracture, can all lead to frozen shoulder. The reason could be prolonged immobilization of the shoulder joint due to referred pain, etc.

Pathology

- During abduction, and repeated overhead activities of the shoulder, long head of biceps and rotator cuff undergo repeated strain. This results in inflammation, fibrosis and consequent thickening of the shoulder capsule, which results in loss of movements (Figs 2.2A and B). *If the movements are continued, then the fibrosis gradually breaks, movements return but never come back to normal.*
- Prolonged activity causes small scapular and biceps muscles to waste faster, load on joint increases and degenerative changes sets in. Capsule is fibrosed and shoulder movements are decreased.

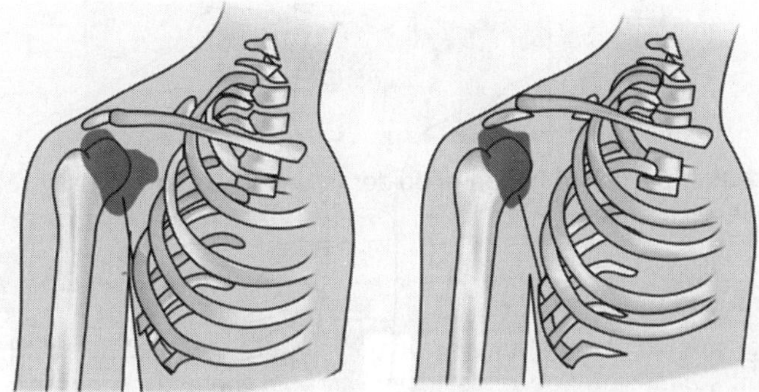

Figs 2.2A and B: (A) Normal capsular pattern, (B) shrinkage of the capsule in frozen shoulder

Clinical Features

A patient with frozen shoulder clinically presents as follows:

- Decreased range of both active and passive shoulder movements.
- The patient demonstrates a capsular pattern of movement restrictions (i.e. external rotation > abduction > internal rotation).
- Pain is noted at the end stage of stretch.

- Accessory joint play is reduced.
- Resistive tests are generally pain free in the available range of motion.
- Patient is unable to do routine daily activities like combing the hair, in case of women wearing the buttons of their blouse, (Fig. 2.3), doing overhead activities, etc.

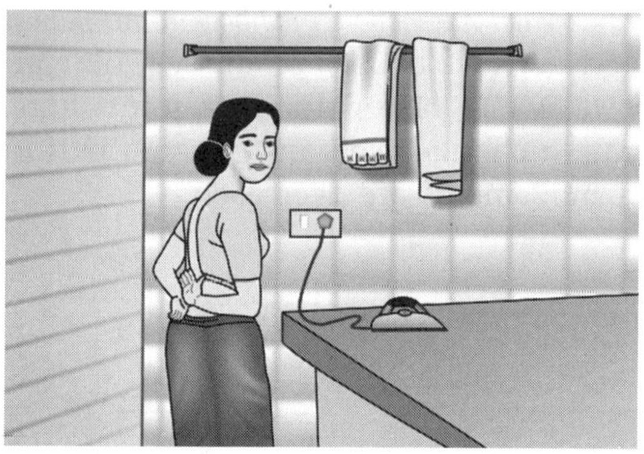

Fig. 2.3: A patient of frozen shoulder is unable to do the daily routine activities like these

Facts you must know

Diagnosis of frozen shoulder is primarily by clinical examination which records capsular type of restriction of both the active and passive range of motion of the shoulder.

Clinical Stages

There are three classical stages in frozen shoulder, according to **Reeves:**

Stage I (stage of pain): Patient complains of acute pain, decreased movements, external rotation greatest followed by loss of abduction and then forward flexion. *Internal rotation is least affected*. This stage lasts for 10–36 weeks.

Note: Pain in frozen shoulder does not radiate below the elbow (Fig. 2.4).

Stage II (stage of stiffness): In this stage, pain gradually decreases and the patient complains of stiff shoulder. Slight movements are present. This lasts for 4–12 months.

Stage III (stage of recovery): Patient will have no pain and movements would have recovered but will never be regained to normal. It lasts for 6 months to 2 years.

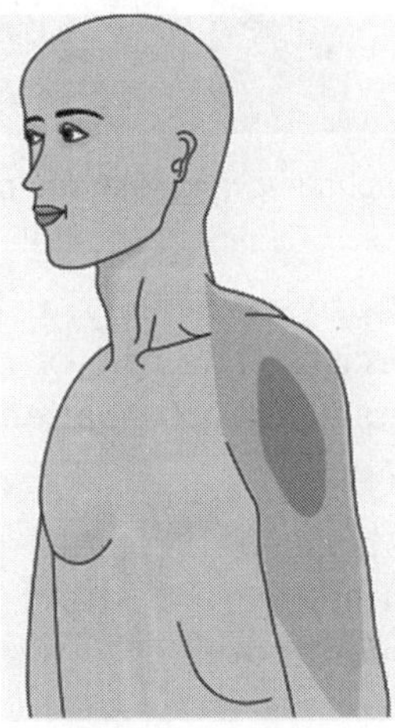

Fig. 2.4: Region of distribution of pain in frozen shoulder

Radiology

X-ray of the shoulder is usually normal; but in a few cases, 'sclerosis' may be seen on the outer edge of greater tuberosity (***Golding's sign***) (Fig. 2.5).

Treatment

Stage I: In this stage, long acting once a day NSAIDs are usually preferred as this condition usually runs a long course (10–36 weeks). Intraarticular steroids may help to provide transient relief of pain only.

Stage II: In this stage, since the pain will have reduced considerably, exercises both active and passive are gradually

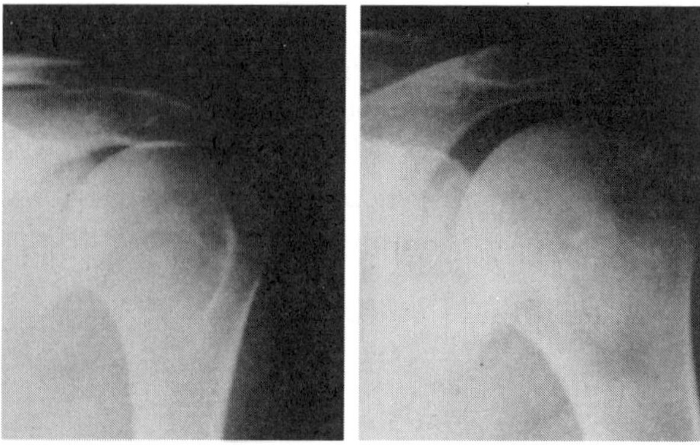

Fig. 2.5: Radiographs showing features of frozen shoulder

begun followed by physiotherapy, ultrasound, heat and shoulder wheel exercises. The role of manipulation of the shoulder is controversial but can be attempted under general anesthesia in this stage.

Stage III: In this stage, active and passive exercises, physiotherapy consisting of short wave diathermy, ultrasound, etc. are continued.

Treatment pearls

- Exercises are most effective than modalities, drugs and steroid injection.
- Mobilization techniques are the other effective method.
- Traditional manipulation under GA is a previous successful method.
- Traditional manipulation under GA is more successful than traction manipulation.
- Arthroscopic distension (Bruisement technique): This helps to increase ROM after several weeks or months.
- *Arthroscopic releases:* This is indicated in recalcitrant cases where the above measures have all failed.

TENNIS ELBOW

I am sure every one is fascinated by tennis. We may not get a place under the sun with Roger Federer, Nadaf, Pete Sampras, Leander Paes, Sania Mirza and others, but certainly, we may get an appointment with an orthopedic surgeon for a problem common in them, that too without playing tennis! Yes, the obvious reference is towards *tennis elbow.*

> *Note:* Sachin Tendulkar should be credited for popularizing and creating lots of awareness and controversies about tennis elbow at least in our country!

History

It was first described from the *Writer's cramps* by Range in 1873. It was Madris who called it as "tennis elbow" shortly thereafter.

Definition

Tennis elbow syndrome encompasses lateral, medial and posterior elbow symptoms. The one commonly encountered is the lateral tennis elbow which is known as the ***classical tennis elbow*** and is the *pain and tenderness on the lateral side of the elbow,* some well-defined and some vague, that results from repetitive stress.

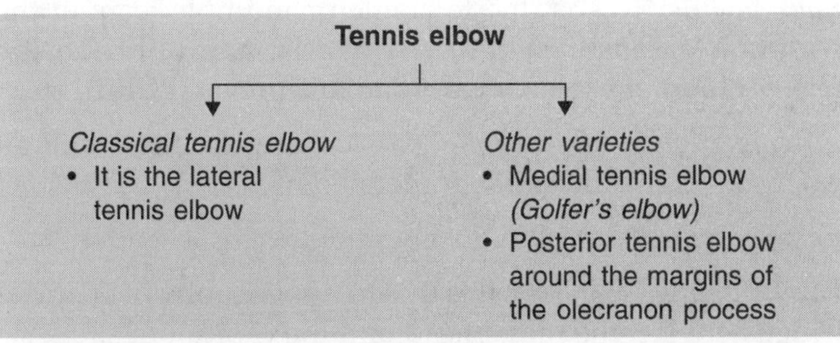

Vital points

Location of pain in tennis elbow

- Lateral epicondyle (75%)
- Lateral muscle mass (17%)
- Medial epicondyle (10%)
- Posterior (8%).

Lateral Tennis Elbow

It is a lesion affecting the tendinous origin of common wrist extensors (Fig. 2.6). It is more common in men than women are and is believed to be a degenerative disorder.

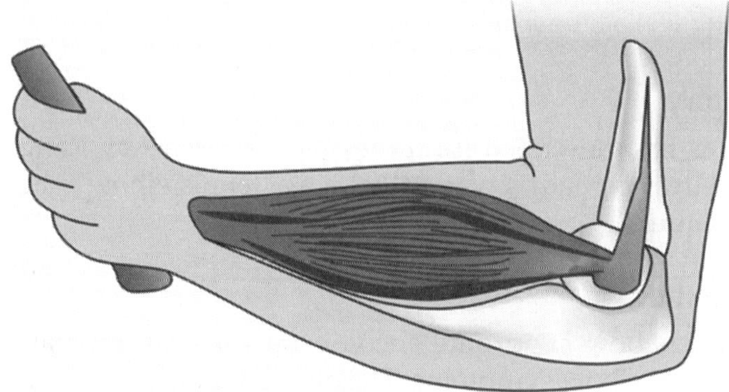

Fig. 2.6: Repetitive stress at common extensor origin in tennis players

Causes

Epicondylitis: This is due to single or multiple tears in the common extensor origin, periostitis, angiofibroblastic proliferation of extensor carpi radialis brevis (ECRB), etc.

Inflammation of adventitious bursa: Between the common extensor origin and radio humeral joint.

Calcified deposits: Within the common extensor tendon.

Painful annular ligament: It is due to hypertrophy of synovial fringe between the radial head and the capitulum's.

Pain of neurological origin, e.g. cervical spine affection, radial nerve entrapment, etc.

Mystifying fact

ECRB is the most commonly involved structure in lateral epicondylitis.

Seen in

- All levels of tennis players.
- In world class players "SERVE" appears to be the cause.
- In less than world class players "backhand stroke".
- Seen in other sports also.
- May be occupational, etc.
- More common in the dominated arm.

Causes in tennis players: More than one-third tennis players all over the world are affected with this problem over 35 years of age.

- Novice
- Playing several games per week.
- More than 35 years of age.
- Equal sex incidence.
- Backhand stroke (38%).
- Serve (25%).
- Forehand stroke (23%).
- Backhand volley (7%).
- Overhead smash (4%).
- Forehand volley (3%).

Contributing factors

- Little playing experience.
- Consistent missing of "*sweet spot*" while hitting.
- Poor stroke techniques: Use of arm instead of body.
- Poor power or flexibility.
- Heavy stiff racket, large handle size, too tight racket stringing.
- Heavy duty wet balls.
- Playing surface—balls bounce quicker off the cement court.

Did you know?

Though called tennis elbow, it is more common in non-tennis players (95%). Causes can be:

- Throwing sports
- Swimming
- Carpentry, plumbing, textile workers
- Housewives

However, up to 50 percent of tennis players suffer from this problem at some time in their sporting career.

Pathophysiology and Related Symptoms

Stage I: There is acute inflammation but no angioblastic invasion. *The patient complains of pain during activity.*

Stage II: This is the stage of chronic inflammation. There is some angioblastic invasion. *The patient complains of pain both during activity and at rest.*

Stage III: Chronic inflammation with extensive angioblastic invasion. *The patient complains pain at rest, night pains, and pain during daily activities.*

Etiology

Problems in tennis players: More than one-third tennis players all over the world are affected with this problem over 35 years of age are obviously due to faculty playing techniques.

Nontennis players: Ironically tennis elbow is more common is nontennis players. This unfortunate group is comprised of housewives, carpenters, miners, drill workers, etc. India's Cricketing Legend Sachin Tendulkar and Sreesanth have made tennis elbow very popular across the country and the world.

Indian housewives: This is the third largest group suffering from this condition. The household chores like washing, brooming, cooking, etc. require repeated extension of the elbow leading to the development of this condition.

Computer related injuries: This is emerging as the recent epidemic among computer professionals across the globe due to repetitive stress while using laptops, mouse, etc.

Clinical Features

Patient complains of pain on the outer aspect of the elbow and has difficulty in gripping objects and lifting them. Sportspersons will have difficulty in extending the elbow. The following are some of the useful clinical tests.

Clinical Tests

Local tenderness on the outside of the elbow at the common extensor origin with aching pain in the back of the forearm (Fig. 2.7).

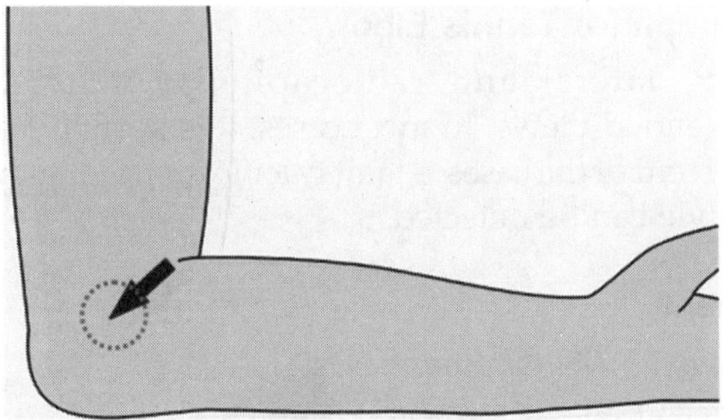

Fig. 2.7: Arrow showing site of tenderness in tennis elbow

Cozen's test: Painful resisted extension of the wrist with elbow in full extension elicits pain at the lateral elbow (Fig. 2.8).

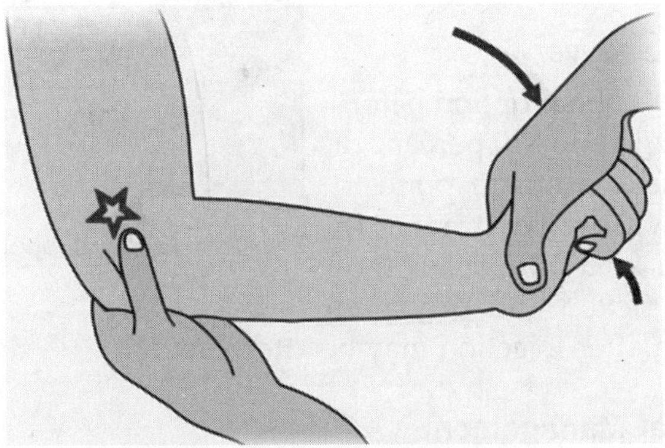

Fig. 2.8: Method of performing the Cozen's test

Elbow held in extension, passive wrist flexion and pronation produces pain.

Maudsley's test: Resisted extension of the middle finger (Remember the letter 'M') elicits pain at the lateral epicondyle due to disease in the extensor digitorum communis.

Radiograph for Tennis Elbow

The AP, lateral and radiocapitellar views are the recommended views. In most cases, it is normal. However, in 16 percent of the cases, a faint calcification along the lateral epicondyle can be detected.

Treatment

Conservative Management

It consists of rest and physiotherapy. In tennis players exercises, light racket, smaller grip, elbow strap, etc. are helpful (Fig. 2.9). Injection of local anesthetic and steroid are useful in 40 percent of cases.

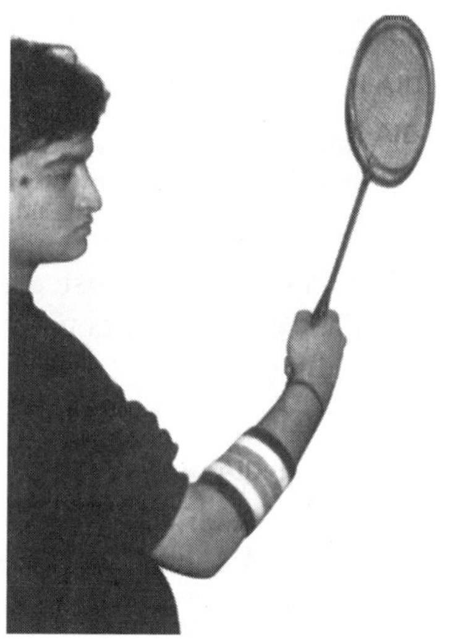

Fig. 2.9: Elbow supports to be used in tennis elbow

Mill's Maneuver

This is the final option before surgery. About 10 percent of the cases do not respond to conservative treatment. In them, a forceful extension of a fully flexed and pronated forearm after injection may be attempted.

Surgical Management

Indications

- Severe pain for 6 weeks at least.

- Marked and localized tenderness over lateral epicondyle.
- Failure to respond to restricted activity or immobilization for at least 2 weeks.

Surgical Methods

- Percutaneous release of epicondylar muscles.
- Bosworth technique of excision of the proximal portion of the annular ligament, release of the origin of the extensor muscles, excision of the bursa and excision of synovial fringes.

What is new in the treatment of tennis and golfer's elbow?

- *The use of extracorporeal shock wave therapy (ESWT):* About 2,000 shock waves of 0.04–0.12 nj/mm^2, three times at monthly intervals for 6 months are found to be effective in cases with failed conservative treatment for at least 6 months.
- *Arthroscopic release:* Of ECRB with failed conservative treatment for nearly 6 months. It is minimally invasive and helps in early rehabilitation.
- *Autologous blood injections:* In refractory cases, injections of 2 ml of autologous blood and 0.5 percent bupivicaine has been tried with good success in some centers.
- *Counterforce bracing (called the tennis elbow or forearm band):* These forces release the forces in the ECRB region.
- *Rehabilitative exercises:* These are wrist flexion, extension, forearm supination and pronation, wrist radial and ulnar deviations at three sets of ten repetitions everyday for 2–6 months is known to give good results.
- *Ultrasound-guided percutaneous needle therapy:* This consists of ultrasound-guided corticosteroid injection and needle debridement of the structures around lateral epicondyle.

Indications: In small tears, not responding to conservative therapy and if too small for surgery.

Advantages

- Minimally invasive procedure.
- Restoration of function is rapid.
- The option of surgery is still open.

In expert's hands, it has a success rate of 65 percent.

Quick facts

Significant relief of symptoms in tennis elbow:

• Changing tennis strokes	92 percent
• Stretching exercises	84 percent
• Use of splints	83 percent
• NSAIDs/steroid	85 percent
• Physiotherapy	50–75 percent
• Rest more than 1 month	72 percent

CARPAL TUNNEL SYNDROME

Carpal tunnel syndrome was first described by Sir James Paget in 1854, but the term was coined by Moerisch.

Anatomy

Bones bound the carpal tunnel on three sides and a ligament on one side (Fig. 2.10). The floor is an osseous arch formed by the carpal bones and the transverse carpal ligament forms the roof.

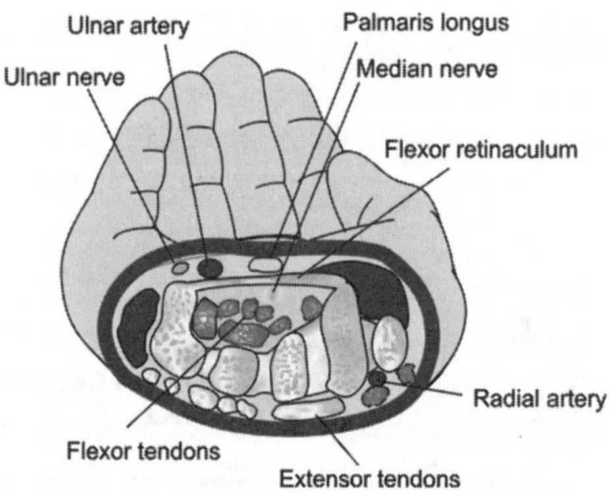

Fig. 2.10: Anatomy of the carpal tunnel

Contents

Tendons of flexor digitorum superficialis and profundus in a common sheath, tendon of flexor pollicis longus in an independent sheath and the median nerve (Fig. 2.11).

Synovitis of the above tendons can generate pressure on the nerve.

Know that 9 tendons and 1 nerve pass through the carpal tunnel.

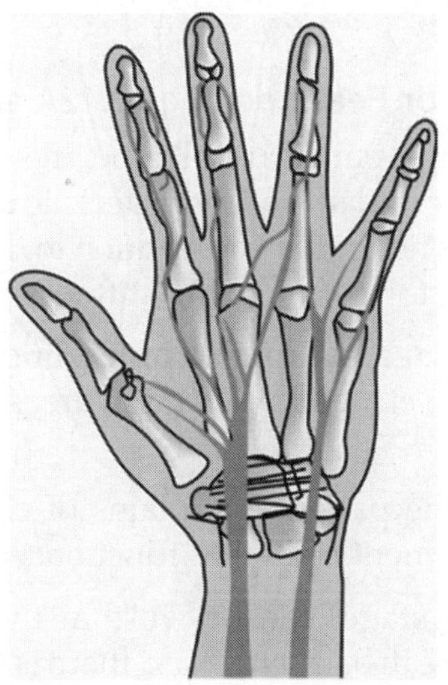

Fig. 2.11: Median nerve coursing through the carpal tunnel

Causes

General

Inflammatory— rheumatoid arthritis.

Endocrine—hypothyroidism, diabetes mellitus, menopause, pregnancy, etc. are some of the important endocrine causes.

Metabolic cause—gout.

Local

These cause crowding of the space. Malunited Colles' fracture, ganglion in the carpal region, osteoarthritis of the carpal bones, and wrist contusion, hematoma, etc. are some of the important local causes.

Remember

Mnemonic PRAGMATIC for causes of carpal tunnel syndrome [(*P*—Pregnancy, *R*—Rheumatoid arthritis, *A*—Arthritis degenerative, *G*—Growth hormone abnormalities (acromegaly), *M*—Metabolic (gout, diabetes myxoedema, etc.), *A*—*Alcoholism*, *T*—Tumors, *I*—Idiopathic, *C*—Connective tissue disorders (e.g. amyloidosis)].

Clinical Stages or Features (Figs 2.12A and B)

Stage I: In this stage, pain is usually the presenting complaint and the patient complains of characteristic discomfort in the hand, but there is no precise localization to the median nerve. There may be history of morning stiffness in the hand.

Stage II: In this stage, symptoms of tingling and numbness, pain, paresthesia, etc. are localized to areas supplied by the median nerve.

Stage III: Here, the patient complains of clumsiness in the hand and impairment of digital functions, etc.

Stage IV: In this stage, sensory loss in the median nerve distribution area can be elicited and there is obvious wasting of the thenar eminence.

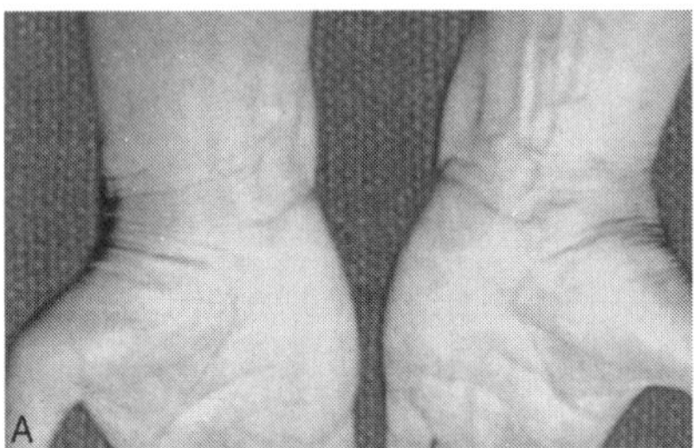

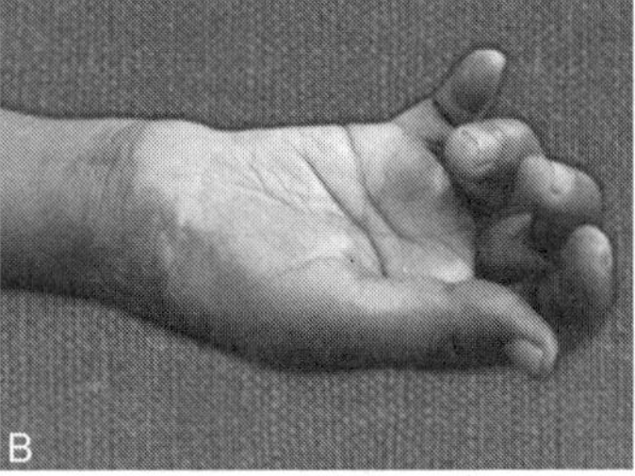

Figs 2.12A and B: (A) Clinical photograph of bilateral carpal tunnel syndrome, (B) Carpal tunnel (clinical photo)

Clinical Tests

These are provocative tests and act as important screening methods and as an adjunct to the electrophysiological testing.

Wrist flexion (Phalen's test): The patient is asked to actively place the wrist in complete but unforced flexion. If tingling and numbness are produced in the median nerve distribution of the hand within 60 seconds, the test is positive. It is the most sensitive provocative test (Fig. 2.13). It has a specificity of 80 percent.

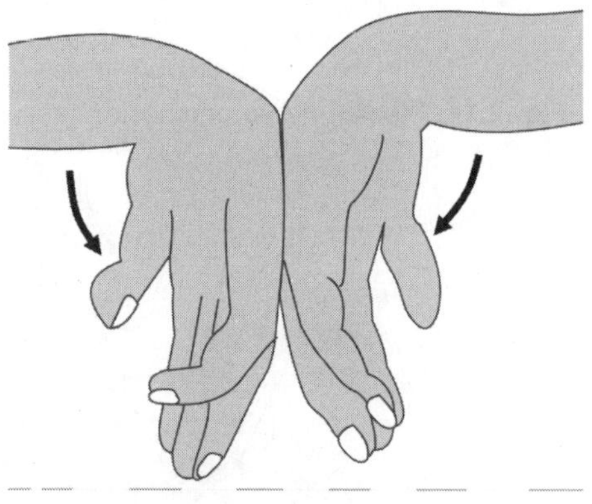

Fig. 2.13: Phalen's test

Tourniquet test: A pneumatic blood pressure cuff is applied proximal to the elbow and inflated higher than the patient's systolic blood pressure. The test is positive if there is paresthesia or numbness in the region of median nerve distribution of the hand. It is less reliable and is specific in 65 percent of cases only.

Median nerve percussion test: The examiner gently taps the median nerve at the wrist (Fig. 2.14). The test is positive if there is tingling sensation. Seen only in 45 percent of cases.

Median nerve compression test: Direct pressure is exerted equally over both wrists by the examiner (Fig. 2.15). The first phase of the test is the time taken for symptoms to appear (15 sec to 2 min). The second phase is the time taken for the symptoms to disappear after release of pressure.

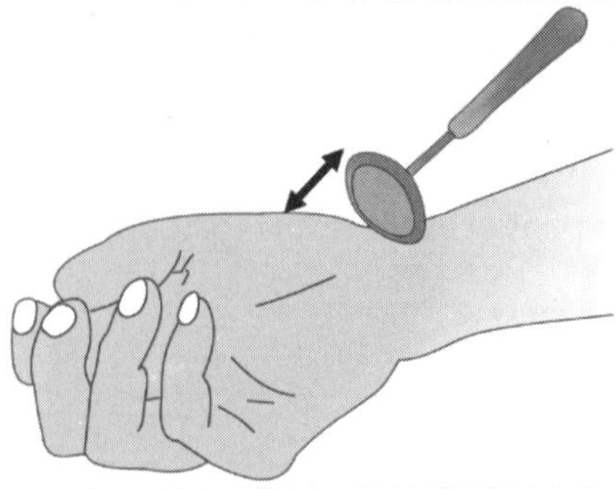

Fig. 2.14: Median nerve percussion test

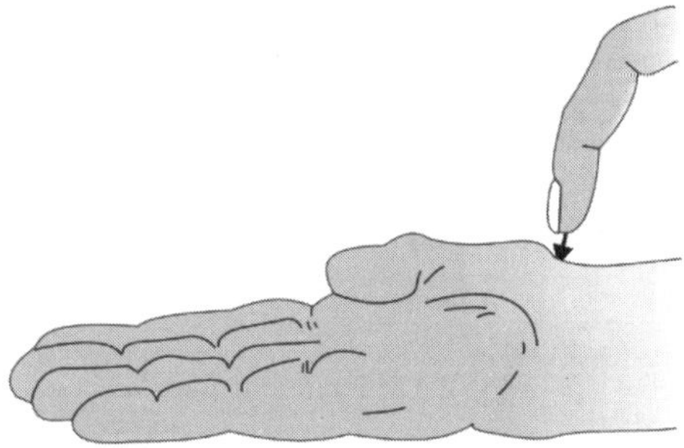

Fig. 2.15: Median nerve compression test

Other Tests

Two-point discrimination test: This test is positive in about one-third cases.

Electrodiagnostic tests are not very infallible with 10 percent individuals having normal values.

Treatment

Nonoperative methods: In the initial stages, non-steroidal anti-inflammatory drugs NSAIDs are given. If it is unsuccessful, steroids like prednisolone for 8 days starting with 40 mg for 2 days and tapering by 10 mg every 2 days are tried. Use of carpal tunnel splint is also advocated (Fig. 2.16).

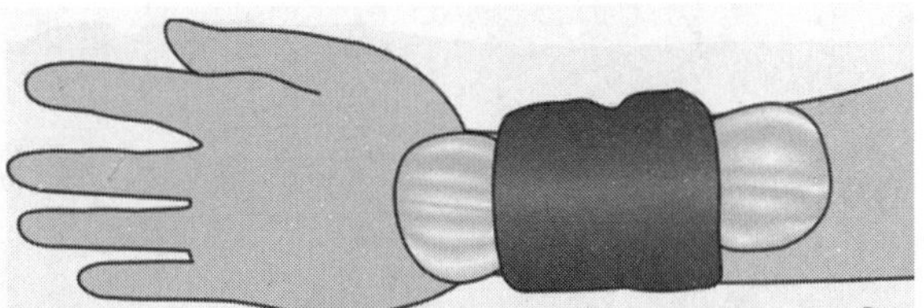

Fig. 2.16: Carpal tunnel splint

Injection treatment: This is indicated in patients with intermittent symptoms, duration of complaints less than one year and if there is no sensory deficits, no marked thenar wasting, etc.

In the injection therapy, a single infusion of cortisone with splinting for 3 weeks is tried.

Surgery: This consists of division of flexor retinaculum and transverse carpal ligament and is indicated in failed nonoperative treatment, thenar atrophy, sensory loss, etc. (Fig. 2.17).

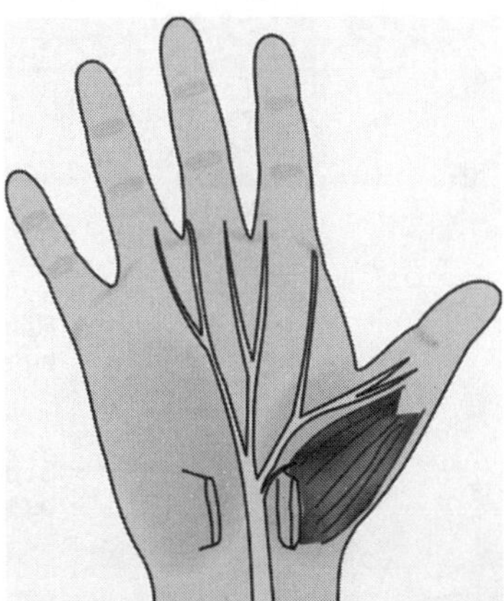

Fig. 2.17: Surgical division of the transverse carpal ligament

What is new in the treatment of carpal tunnel?

Chow's technique

This is an endoscopic release of the carpal ligament. It is a reliable alternative for the open procedure and has a success rate of 93.3 percent.

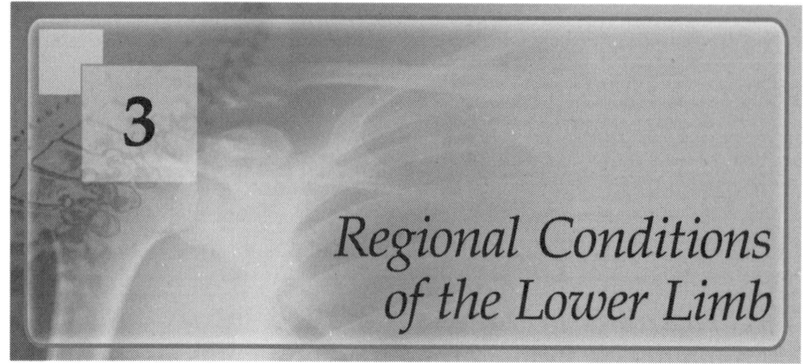

3 Regional Conditions of the Lower Limb

PAINFUL HEEL

The following are some of the causes of pain in the heel (Fig. 3.1)

- Traumatic disturbances.
- Developmental and pathological disturbances.
- Epiphysitis of the calcaneum (Fig. 3.2).

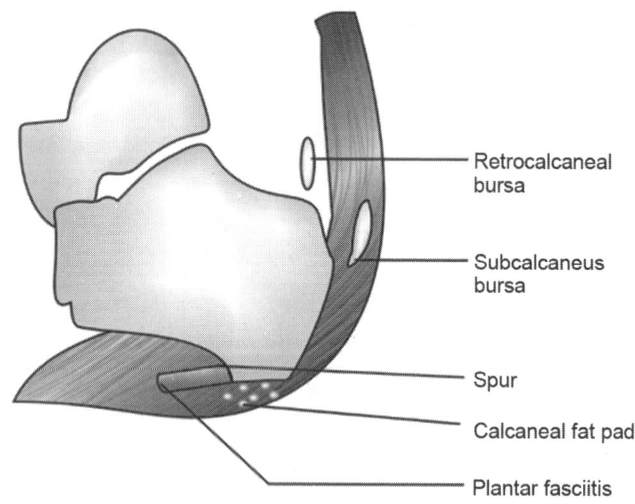

Fig. 3.1: Causes of heel pain

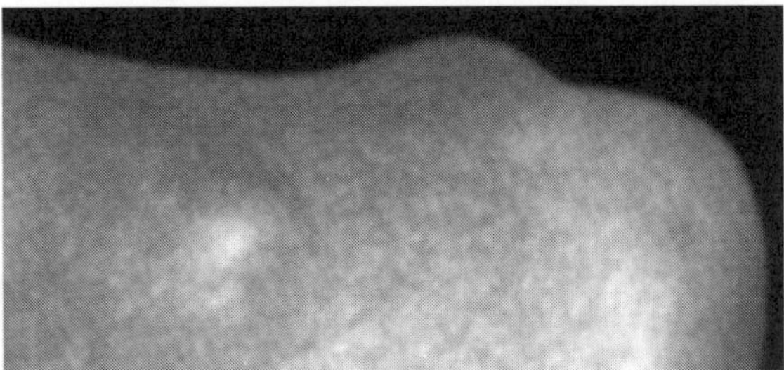

Fig. 3.2: Pump-bump due to friction from the back of the pump shoes (clinical photo)

Differential Diagnosis of Heel Pain

Posterior Heel Pain

- Retrocalcaneal bursitis
- Hageland's deformity (pump-bump)
- Tendo-Achilles or tendonitis
- Calcification within the Achilles tendon
- Referred pain from a soleus muscle triggers point
- Radiculopathy of S_1.

Plantar Heel Pain

- Inflammation or microtrauma of the plantar fascia.
- Entrapping neuropathy of tibial nerve or its branches and sciatic nerve.
- Fat pad atrophy.
- Heel spur.
- Stress fracture of calcaneum.
- Tarsal tunnel syndrome.
- Systemic problems like rheumatoid, etc.
- Radiculopathy of S_1.
- Irritates of the first branch of lateral plantar nerve or nerve to abductor digiti minimi (Baxter's nerve).
- Plantar heel bursitis.
- Thrombosis of the plantar medial venous plexus.
- Post-traumatic fat pad insufficiency (after due to calcaneal fracture).

PLANTAR FASCIITIS (Subcalcaneal Pain)

This is defined as pain on the plantar surface of the heel and is the most common cause of posterior heel pain (Fig. 3.3).

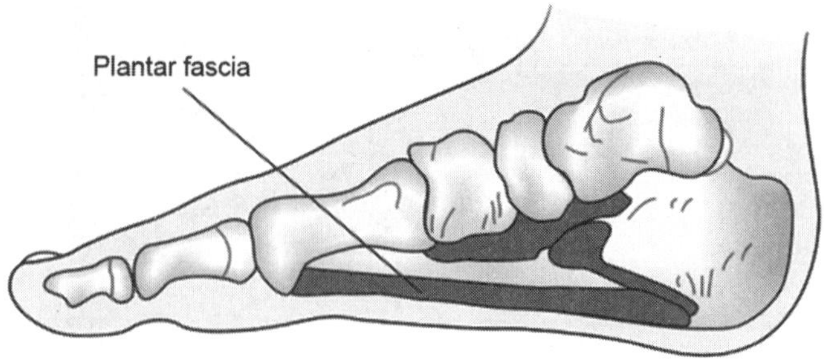

Fig. 3.3: Plantar fascia

Do you know the source of pain in plantar fasciitis?

- Plantar fascia
- Subcalcaneal bursa
- Fat pad
- Tendinous insertion of the intrinsic muscles
- Long plantar ligament
- Medial calcaneal branch of tibial nerve
- Nerve to abductor digiti minimi

Clinical Features

The patient complains of pain in the heel, which is more in the morning. It gradually subsides as the patient takes a few steps. The pain increases on prolonged standing, walking, etc.

Clinical Tests

Tenderness can be elicited on the medial aspect of the posterior heel. Passive stretching of the toes increases pain in the heel (Figs 3.4A and B).

Mystifying facts: Why is plantar heel pain more in the morning?

During sleep, foot is in plantar flexed position causing shortening of the plantar structures. Sudden dorsiflexion in waking up from the night's sleep stretches the structured abruptly causing pain.

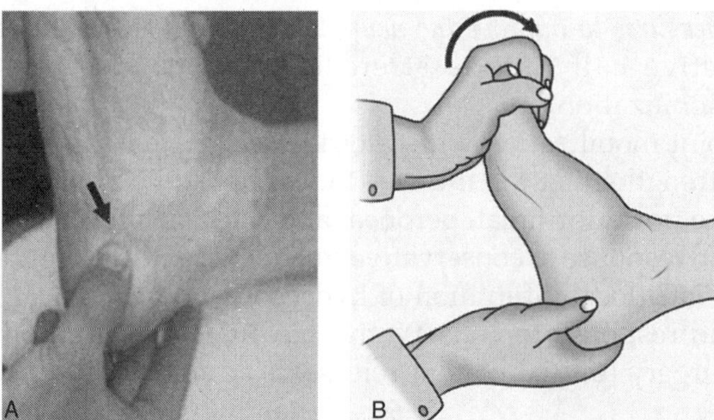

Figs 3.4A and B: (A) Method of eliciting tenderness in plantar fasciitis, (B) Passive stretching of toes increases pain

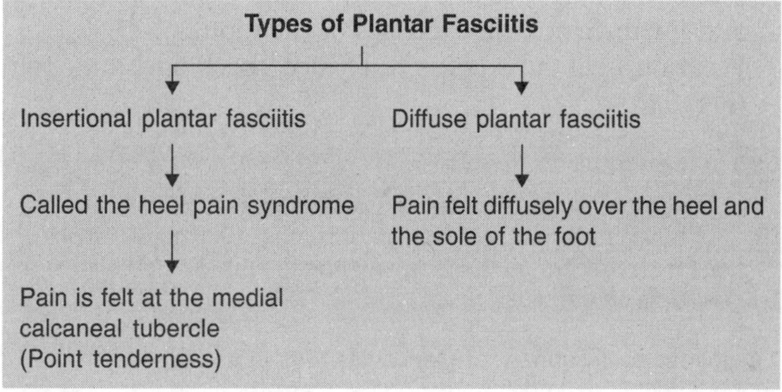

Radiographs

Consisting of the routine AP, lateral and oblique views is advised. However, the X-ray does not show any changes in plantar fasciitis. It helps to detect calcaneal spur and other heel pathologies.

Treatment

- *Measures to reduce pain and inflammation* taping, temporary or permanent shoe orthosis, heel cushion, weight management, etc.

- *Measures to improve the neurodynamics of the tibial nerve*—active calf muscle stretching and calf soft tissue mobilization.
- Joint mobilization with talocalcaneal glides.
- Strengthening the muscles that support the arch namely the posterior tibial, peroneal and intrinsic muscles.
- No response to conservative treatment for three months—LIHC (local infiltration of hydrocortisone) is indicated.
- No response to conservative treatment for 6 months—surgery (partial plantar release) is advised.

Rehabilitation Methods

- Massage the heel by hand.
- Rolling of the foot over a tennis ball.
- Stretching exercises of the tendo-Achilles and hamstrings and intrinsic muscle exercises of the foot.
- Wearing heel cups helps to reduce shock and thus pain (Fig. 3.6).

What is new?

- Endoscopic plantar fasciotomies have a success rate of 85 percent.
- For recalcitrant heel pain instead of surgery 1000 impulses of low energy extracorporeal shock wave treatment (3 applications) is found to be effective.

Quick facts: Treatment of plantar fasciitis in a nutshell

I line

- NSAIDs.
- Heel pad/cushion.
- Stretching exercises of the ankle and foot.

II line

- Local infiltration of hydrocortisone.
- Custom moulded foot orthosis.
- Soft supportive shoes.
- Foot strapping.
- Stretching exercises.
- Night brace or AFO or short leg walking cast.

III line

Surgery if the entire regime mentioned above fail after one year.

CALCANEAL SPURS

It is a spike of bone at the anterior edge of the calcaneal tuberosity (usually medial).

It may be seen on the posterior aspect of the calcaneum also and is called the retrocalcaneal spur (Fig. 3.5).

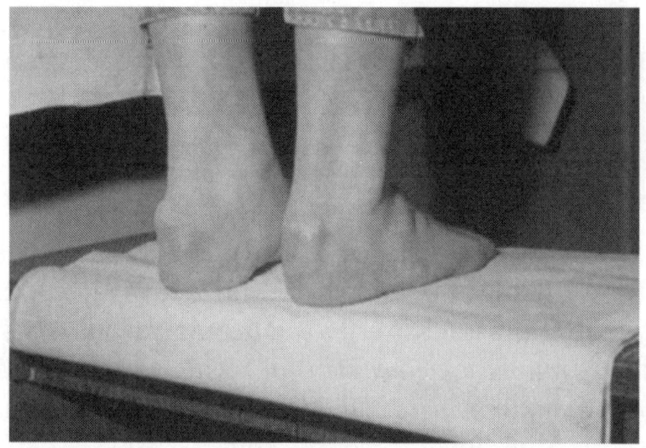

Fig. 3.5: Retrocalcaneal spur (clinical photo)

Causes

- Due to repeated attacks of plantar fasciitis.
- Due to repeated trauma.
- Constant pulls of the shortened plantar fascia.
- Ill-fitting footwear (Figs 3.6A and B).
- Fibromatosis of the plantar fascia.

Important spur facts

- Nearly 80 percent of patients with plantar fasciitis have plantar heel spurs.
- About 10 percent of the general population has asymptomatic heel spurs.
- Though believed, it is actually not the source of pain.
- Many patients with "suspected painful heel spur syndrome" have actually plantar fasciitis.
- Spur has no therapeutic or prognostic significance.

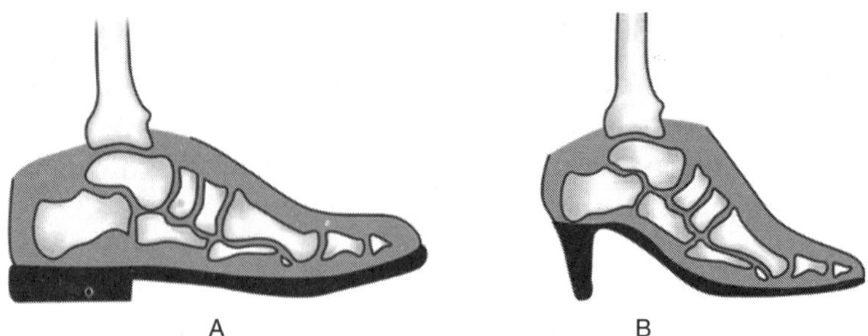

Figs 3.6A and B: (A) Correct footwear, (B) Improper footwear which distorts the normal arches of the foot

Clinical Features

The patient complains of pain over ball of the heel, tenderness on plantar aspect of the heel (Fig. 3.7), slight swelling at the attachment of plantar fascia. *It is due to fibrositis or traumatic detachment of plantar fascia and does not give rise to symptoms per se and the pain when present is due to the causative condition and not the spur.*

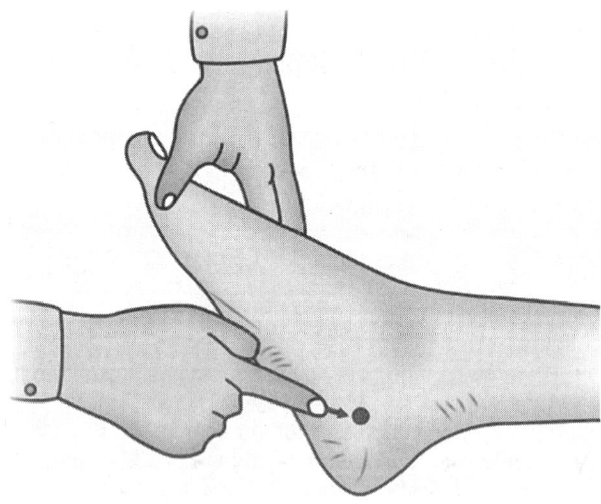

Fig. 3.7: Point of tenderness in plantar fasciitis and calcaneal spur

Radiographs

Lateral view of the heel show prominent bone spike arising from the calcaneum (Fig. 3.8).

Pitfall: Only 50 percent of the patient with heel pain show calcaneal spurs on X-ray.

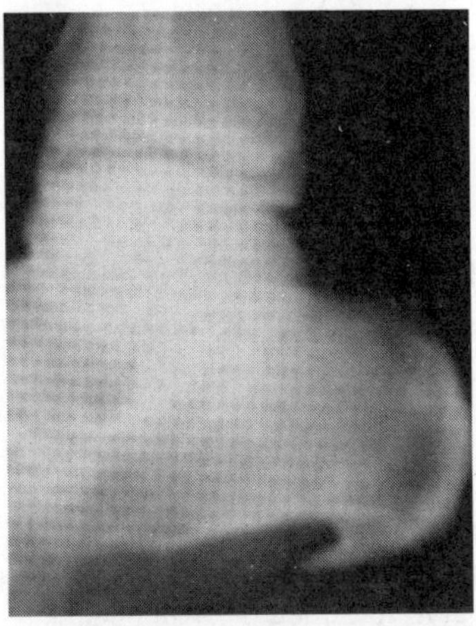

Fig. 3.8: Radiograph showing calcaneal spur (best seen in the lateral view)

Treatment

Conservative methods include treating the causative factor, rest, NSAIDs, local infiltration of hydrocortisone and microcellular rubber (MCR) used for the sole of the footwear (Fig. 3.9).

Surgery is indicated when no relief is seen with the conservative treatment.

Methods

- Osteotomy of the calcaneus.
- Decompressing operation with multiple drill holes in the calcaneus.
- Excision of the medial inferior tuberosity.

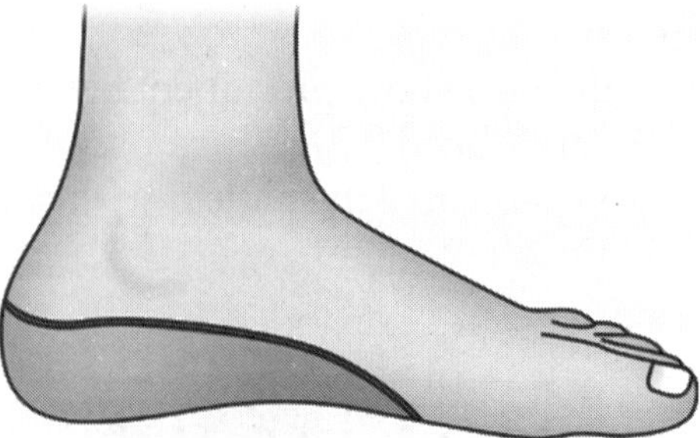

Fig. 3.9: UC-BL shoe inserts to relieve heel stress in plantar fasciitis and calcaneal spur

What is new in the the treatment of calcaneal spur?

- Endoscopic treatment of calcaneal spur syndrome.
  Indications: Recalcitrant heel pain.
  Procedure: Medial endoscopy and lateral instrumentation.
  - Debridement of posterior roof of the calcaneal arch.
  - Removal of calcaneal spurs.
  - Lateral to medial release of plantar fascia.
  - Debridement of the periosteum of calcaneal tuberosity.
  - Release of nerve to abductor digiti minimi.
- Low-dose acoustic shock waves delivered by a machine called an Ossatron. The acoustic waves may work by stimulating increased blood flow to the area, decrease inflammation and help the tissue to heel.

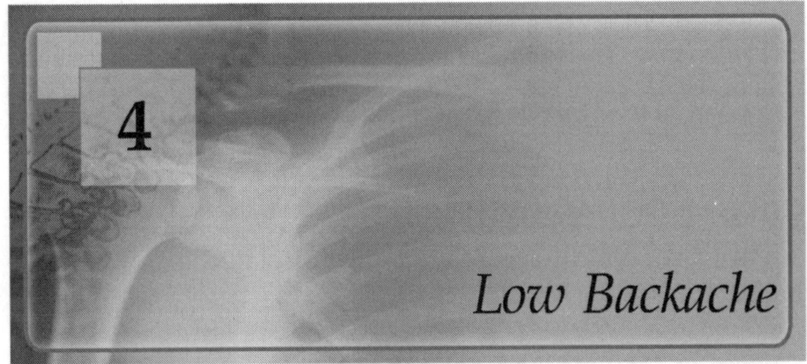

APPROACH TO A PATIENT WITH LOW BACKACHE

Low backache is an extremely common malady afflicting the human race across the globe cutting the geographical boundaries, race, culture, etc. Eighty to ninety percent of the human population will suffer from some form of backache, mild or severe in their lifetime. It is of interest to know the historical background regarding low back pain.

Historical review

- Backache and leg pain are known since beginning of history.
- Primitive culture called it a work of a demon.
- Greeks recognized the symptoms as disease.
- In the 18th century, Cotumis attributed pain to the sciatic nerve.
- In 1881, Lasegue test described a test to distinguish hip disease from sciatica (first described by Frost).
- Virchow Kocher, etc. described acute traumatic ruptures of the disk that resulted in death.
- Goldthwait (1911) first attributed back pain to posterior displacement of disk.
- Dandy (1929) first reported removal of a disk tumor from patients suffering from sciatica.
- Myelography was first described in 1922.
- Barr (1932) finally attributed the source of sciatica to the herniated lumbar disk.
- Barr (1934) suggested surgical treatment for disk excision.
- Layman Smith (1963) suggested enzymatic dissolution of disk.

- Kirkaldy-Willis opine aging as the primary theory in disk disease.
- Nuchenson in 1964, White and Punjabi in 1982 described biomechanics of spine.
- Schnack in 1983 described clinical anatomy.

CAUSES OF BACKACHE

A variety of conditions related and unrelated to spine cause backache (*see the box*).

Common Causes of Backache

The common causes of backache are:

Unaccustomed activities: A sedentary person suddenly adopting an active form of life, etc.

Poor posture: Improper posture during sitting, walking, standing, and working places, enormous load on the back and results in backache. *This is by far the most common cause of low backache* (Figs 4.1A to F).

Occupational backache: Certain occupation places enormous stress on the back, e.g. garbage collectors, porters.

Obesity: Protruding abdomen places enormous strain on the back.

Muscle strain: In 80 percent of the cases, backache is due to sprain of the back muscles during activity, sports, trauma, etc.

Prolapsed lumbar intervertebral disk: This is the second most common cause for low back pain after muscle strain and ligament sprain. Discussed at great length in the previous section.

The facet joint osteoarthritis due to old age, repeated bending and twisting activities lead to arthritis of facet joints.

Spinal stenosis: Spinal stenosis due to degenerative process is another common cause.

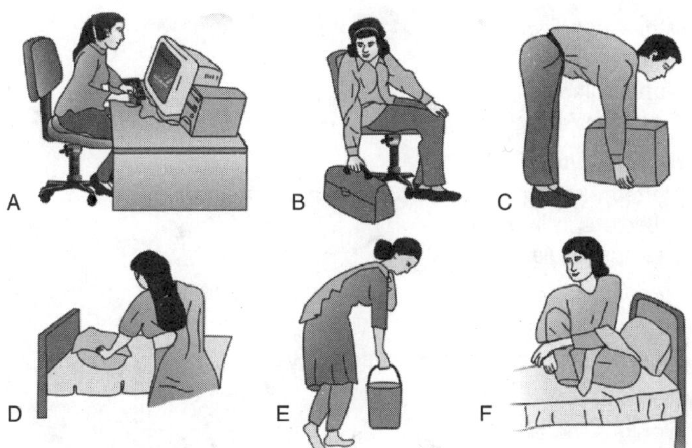

Figs 4.1A to F: Various common mechanisms of acute low backache: (A) Improper posture, (B) Sudden twist, (C) Faulty weightlifting, (D) Bending, (E) Sudden weightlifting, (F) Faulty sitting

Uncommon Causes of Backache

Uncommon causes of backache are diseases of the spine, fractures, tumors, inflammatory conditions, etc.

Quick Facts: Causes of low backache (Fig. 4.2)

Common causes

- Back muscle sprain
- Prolapsed lumbar intervertebral disk
- Obesity
- Poor posture
- Facet joint arthritis
- Unaccustomed activities
- Occupational causes

Uncommon causes

Congenital causes (4 'S')

- Scoliosis
- Spondylolisthesis
- Spina bifida
- Spondylolysis

Infective conditions
- Osteomyelitis
- Tuberculosis
- Brucellosis, etc.

Traumatic causes
- Vertebral body injuries, posterior arch fractures
- Muscle sprain/strain
- Prolapsed disk

Inflammatory causes
- Rheumatoid arthritis
- Ankylosing spondylitis and other SSAs

Neoplasm
- Benign—osteoid osteoma
- Malignant—secondary, multiple myeloma, etc.

Metabolic causes
- Osteoporosis
- Osteomalacia

Degenerative conditions
- Osteoarthritis
- Lumbar spondylosis

Referred pain from
- Gynecological diseases
- Genitourinary diseases
- Gastrointestinal conditions, etc.

Presenting Complaints

Age: Backache is more common in middle-aged and elderly people (usually degenerative). In young adults, it is due to trauma; and in children, it is usually due to organic lesions.

Age predilection and low backache

Age common causes
- < 20 years Spondylolysis
- 20-40 years Disk herniation
- > 40 years Spondylosis
  Lumbar canal stenosis

Common to all age groups:
Ligament sprain/muscle strains.

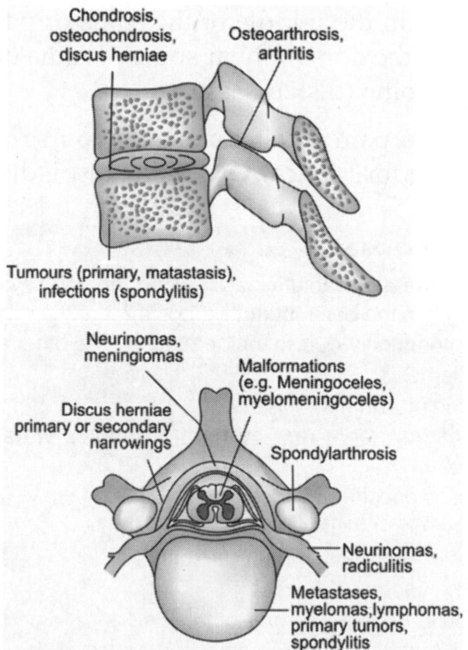

Fig. 4.2: Causes of uncommon low backache and pathological processes of the spine, which can give rise to local spinal pain syndromes associated with painful muscle spasms

Sex: Osteoporosis, rheumatoid arthritis, etc. are more common in females. Ankylosing spondylitis, trauma, secondary, etc. are more common in males.

Occupation: People with sedentary jobs and heavy manual laborers are frequently prone for backache.

Pain

Over 90 percent of the patients complain of pain in the lower back. The following points should be enquired:

Nature of pain: Is it sudden (trauma) or gradual (spondylosis)? Did weightlifting, sudden bending, etc. precede it? Is there remissions and exacerbations (disk disease) or is it continuous (tumors)? Is there history of night cries (e.g. TB spine)? Does rest relieve it? Does it radiate to the lower limbs? etc.

Site: Is the pain in the middle of the spine or paravertebral muscles. Is it in the dorsolumbar spine (trauma or tumor) or in the lumbar spine (disk disease)?

Sciatic pain: Here, pain radiates along the course of the sciatic nerve (see causes for sciatica). Common cause is disk prolapse.

Sciatica and its causes

Sciatica is defined as a radiating pain along the course of the sciatic nerve and is felt in the back, buttocks, posterior of the thigh, legs and the foot. It is commonly due to disk prolapse. The other causes are:

- Spondylolisthesis.
- Sacroiliac joint arthritis.
- Affliction of the nerve root by herpes simplex virus can cause radicular pain.
- Tuberculoma causing cord compression.
- Lymphomas and pelvic malignancy.
- Incurled thickened ligamentum flavum.
- Cysts of the sacral nerve root.
- Intraspinal neurofibromas and other tumors.
- Hemorrhage in the ependymoma can cause sudden and gross neurological deficit, mimicking acute disk prolapse.
- Diabetic neuropathy, etc.

Biochemical Causes

Recently, it has been suggested but not clearly demonstrated that blood pooling in various blood vessels surrounding the nerve roots may contribute to impaired nerve root formation and sciatica.

Neurogenic Claudication

This is a feature of spinal canal stenosis.

Neurological Symptoms

These consist of paresthesia, muscle weakness, disturbance of sphincters, cauda equina syndrome, etc.

Facet Syndromes

Here, the patient complains of chronic backache, early morning stiffness, difficulty in getting out of bed, standing, sitting or climbing.

Other Complaints

There may be history of stiffness, pain in other joints (e.g. rheumatoid arthritis), constitutional symptoms (e.g. tuberculosis, malignancy), genitourinary complaints, etc.

Physical Signs

Stance and gait: Does the patient stand with a normal stance or has deformities like scoliosis, kyphosis, lordosis or pelvic tilt. Is the gait normal or altered?

Spasm: This is seen in acute painful conditions of the spine. The patient complains of pain in the Para vertebral muscles and painful restriction of all the spine movements.

Movements: There may be restriction of the spine movements due to the organic lesions affecting the back.

Swelling: Swelling due to cold abscesses may be present.

Tenderness: It may be present over the spinous process, in between the spinous processes, over muscles, ligaments, facet joints, etc.

Neurological Examination

This consists of examinations of the various dermatomes for sensations, myotomes for muscle power and reflexes (*see* pages 62 and 63).

SLRT and tension signs: This is to know the effects of disk prolapse on the sciatic nerve (the tests are described on (*see* page 61).

Other Examinations

Other exar ... acent joints, perip ... ginal examinatio

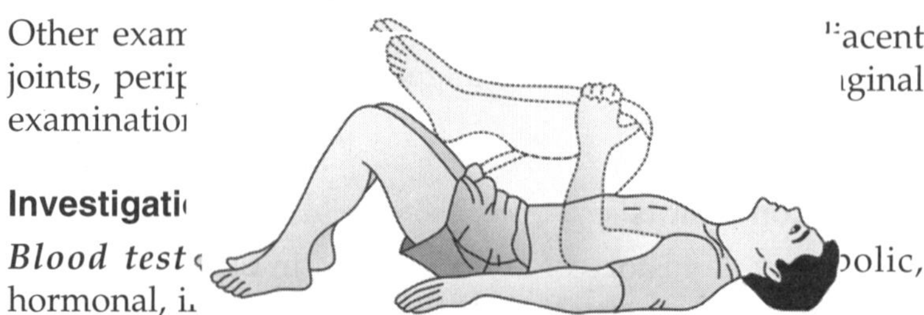

Investigati

Blood test ... bolic, hormonal, i

Radiology: Routine plain radiographs of the lumbar spine are advised. Both anteroposterior and lateral views are usually required. Oblique views are helpful in detecting the fracture of pars. Though X-rays are not very helpful in detecting the disk prolapse, it is of value in diagnosing metabolic, degenerative, inflammatory, malignant conditions affecting the spine.

Myelography: This procedure is not routinely used anymore because of its complications. However, it has a role in demonstrating blocks due to disk prolapse.

CT scan: It is a noninvasive procedure and helps to identify the bone and soft tissue problems with greater accuracy.

MRI scan: This is the gold standard in the investigations of the spine. It is noninvasive and is better than CT scan in diagnosing the bone and soft tissue problems around the spine. However, its high cost is prohibitive and is available only in major cities and centers.

Treatment

The underlying cause has to be detected and managed accordingly. The treatment for backache consists of drugs like NSAIDs, muscle relaxants, physiotherapy, traction, use of belts and corsets (Fig. 4.3). Proper postural habits, back exercises and back education go a long way in preventing the backache. Surgery is done for specific indications (*see* pages 75 to 77).

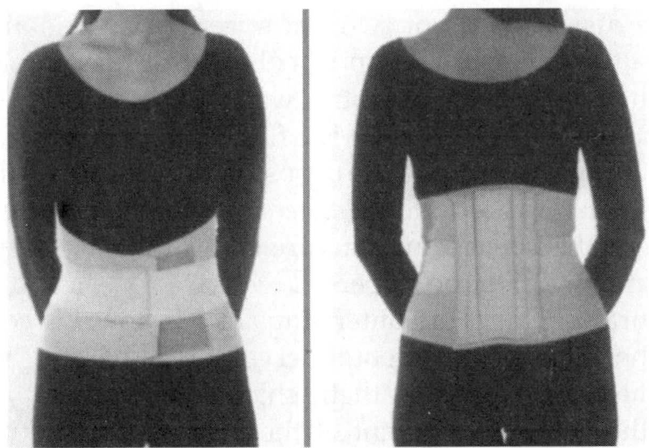

Figs 4.3: Lumbar sacral belt application in LBA

LUMBAR DISK DISEASE AND DISK PROLAPSE

Disk Anatomy

Development of spine starts from the third week of intrauterine life and continues until third decade of life. There are 23 disks throughout the spine, absent only in atlantoaxial articulation. It is thinnest in the thoracic region and thickest in the lumbar. Each disk is interposed between the bodies of a pair of vertebrae. Body of each vertebra is covered by a thin end plate of a bone, which is perforated by numerous tiny holes. This in turn is covered by a hyaline cartilage, which may be considered as the outermost portion of the disk.

Anteriorly and laterally, the bodies and the disks are bounded firmly by the anterior longitudinal ligament and posteriorly by the posterior longitudinal ligament, which is weak. The intervertebral disks in adults are avascular; the cells within it are sustained by diffusion of nutrients into the disk through the pores in the bodies. Movements and weightbearing help in diffusion. Degeneration of the disk may be prompted by changes in the permeability of the cartilage end plate.

The disk consists of two parts; centrally, it is *nucleus pulposus, which* is made-up of collagen fibrils, fibrocytes, chondrocytes, gelatinous matrix, water and salt. Peripherally, it has *annulus fibrosus, which* is a fibrocartilaginous tissue. It is thick anteriorly and thin posteriorly more so in the posterolateral aspect. *Hence, posterolateral disk prolapse is more common*. The fibers of annulus are joined by diagonal fibers also known as Sharpe's fibers.

Neural fibers in the outer rings of the annulus contain branches of the sinovertebral nerve dorsally and ventrally branches from the sympathetic chain.

With age, water content of the disk decreases, fibrous tissue and cartilage cells increase, and the nucleus becomes granular and friable.

Mystifying facts about the disks

- There is no disk between C_1 and C_2
- It is avascular and gets its nutrition through local diffusion
- The nutrition of the disk is best in side lying position
- 80 percent of the nutrition process takes place in the first one hour of night's rest
- The outer annulus fibrosus of the disk is innervated by the sinovertebral nerve and gray ramus communicants of the sympathetic chain.

DISK PHYSIOLOGY

Disk apart from giving the spine its mobility functions as a shock absorber. Following loss of disk, the vertebral body reacts to abnormal pressure forces by hypertrophy bone formation at the surface revealed as sclerosis and osteophyte formation. Schmorl's node is the disk material, which has escaped into the body through the pores and is walled off by the fibrous tissue.

What is the Natural History of Lumbar Disk Disease?

All spines degenerate with advancing age and so does the intervertebral disks. Degenerative process is divided into three stages:

Remember

About disk
- It gives spine the mobility.
- It acts as a shock absorber.
- It is fibrocartilaginous.
- It increases the height of the spine by 25 percent.
- Centrally, it has a nucleus pulposus and peripherally annulus fibrosus.
- It is avascular.
- Annulus fibers are weak posteriorly; hence, posterolateral disk prolapse is more common.
- With age, water content of the disk falls.

Stage of dysfunction
- Seen between 15 and 45 years of age.
- Circumferential and radial tears are seen in the disk annulus.
- Localized synovitis of the facet joints is seen.

Stage of instability
- Seen between 35 and 70 years of age.
- There is an internal disruption of the disk.
- Progressive disk resorption takes place.
- Degeneration of facet joints with lax capsules, subluxation and joint erosions are seen.

Stage of stabilization
- Seen over 60 years of age.
- Progressive development of hypertrophic bone about the disk and facet joints leading to segmental stiffening or frank ankylosis is seen.

Disk herniation is considered as a complication of disk degeneration in stages II and I (Fig. 4.4). Spinal stenosis is a complication in late instability and early stabilization stages. Disk can herniate either into the body as Schmorl's node or posteriorly towards the canal compressing the nerve roots.

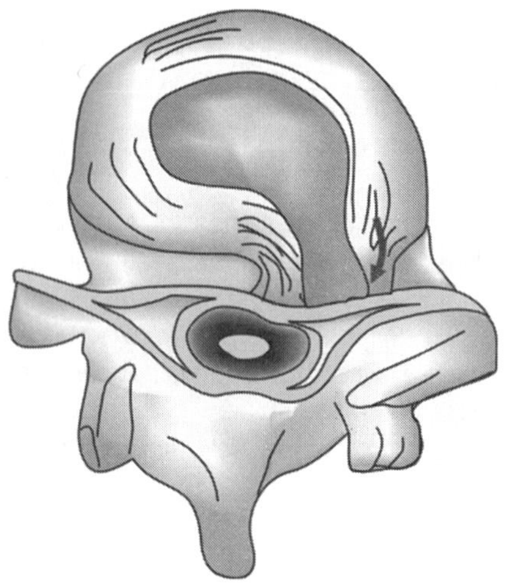

Fig. 4.4: Posterolateral disk herniation

Classification of Prolapsed Intervertebral Disk

(Fig. 4.5) (For medical readers only)

Disk bulging or protrusion: This refers to some eccentric accumulation of nucleus with slight deformity of the annulus.

Prolapsed disk is the one in which eccentric nucleus produces a definite deformity as it works through the fibers of the annulus.

Extruded disk: Here, the disk comes out into the canal and impinges on the adjacent nerve root (Fig. 4.6).

Sequestrated disk: Here the nuclear material has separated from the disk itself and potentially migrates.

Interesting facts

Do you know at what levels lumbar disk prolapse most commonly occur does?

$L_{4-5} > L_5S_1 > L_{3-4} > L_{2-3} > L_{1-2}$

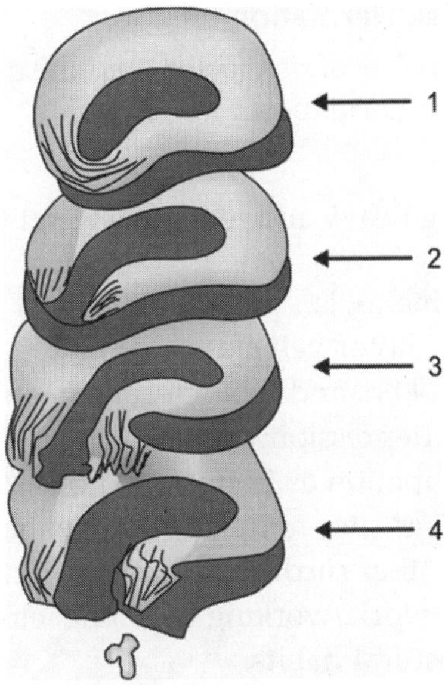

Fig. 4.5: Types of prolapse disk: (1) Bulge disk, (2) Prolapse disk, (3) Extruded disk, and (4) Sequestrated disk

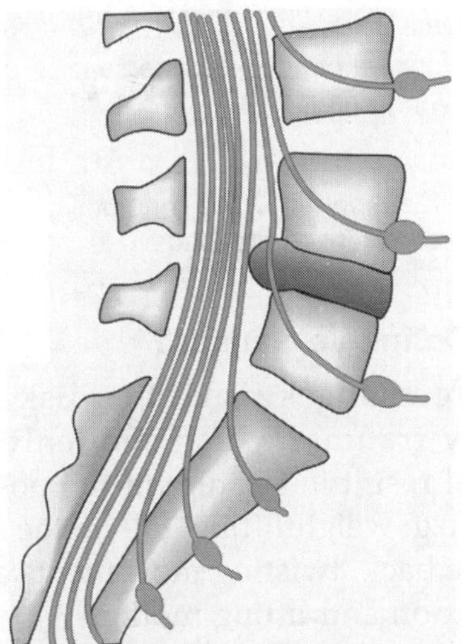

Fig. 4.6: Disk prolapse compressing the nerve root

Etiology of Disk Herniation

The etiology consists of risk factors and the definitive causes resulting in disk herniation.

Risk factors

- Jobs requiring heavy and repetitive weightlifting (Figs 4.7 and 4.8).
- Use of machine tools.
- Operation of motor vehicles.
- Cigarette smokers and tobacco consumers.
- Anxiety and depression.
- Stressful occupation as in doctors, police, etc.
- Women with greater number of pregnancies.
- Obesity and other cardiovascular risk factors.
- Monotonous work, working overtime, etc.
- Improper postural habits.

Do you know the relative load on your spine measured at L_{3-4}?

- Lying on the sides (25%)
- Standing 100 percent
- Seated 145 percent
- Standing with forward bend — 150 percent
- Sitting with forward bend — 180 percent

Generally

- Load is better in supported sitting than unsupported sitting
- Lumbar support decreases the load.

What are the Definitive Causes?

- Degenerative changes make the disk susceptible to trauma. Any trauma, which suddenly increases the pressure, will result in rupture of the posterior fibers of the annulus, e.g. weightlifting, fall on the buttocks, direct trauma to the back, twisting movements and occupation involving flexion and lifting motions.
- Disk may also rupture during pregnancy, labor and after prolonged bed rest due to disk softening.

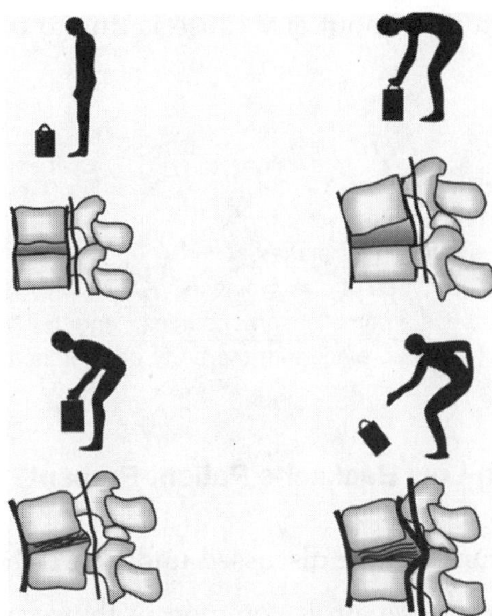

Fig. 4.7: Common mode of disk prolapse due to sudden and improper weightlifting

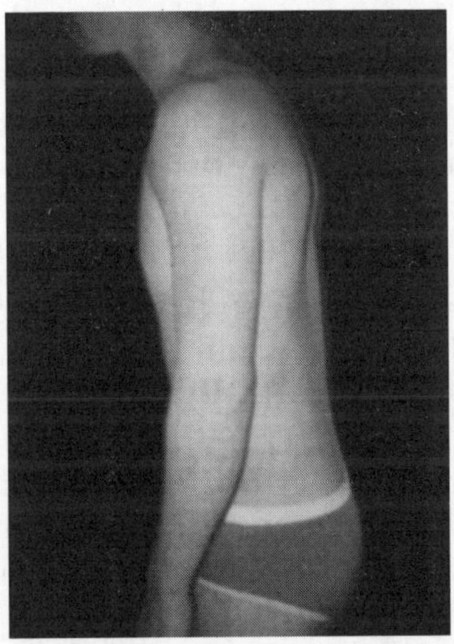

Fig. 4.8: Clinical presentation in a patient with disk slip (clinical photo)

- Disk rupture without any cause is due to degenerative process.

Remember

About disk disease

- It is due to aging process.
- It passes through three stages.
- There are four types of disk prolapse.
- Disk prolapse is a complication of stages I and II.
- Herniation can take place into the body or posteriorly into spinal canal.

How Does a Low Backache Patient Present? Clinical Features

Clinical features can be discussed under three headings:

Low backache: Back pain is common in the second decade, disk disease and disk herniation in the third or fourth decade. *The usual history of lumbar disk herniation is of repetitive low back pain, radiating to the buttocks and decreased by rest.* Pain is increased by flexion episode, sitting, straining, sneezing, coughing, etc. Pain is decreased by rest and in semi-Fowler position.

Radiculopathy: This refers to pain in the distribution of the sciatic nerve and is invariably due to disk herniation. This is called as sciatica. *Leg pain equal to or more than the back pain evidence the radicular pain from the nerve root compression due to herniated disk.* Pain usually begins in the lower back radiating to the sacroiliac regions, buttocks and thigh. The radicular pain usually extends below the knee.

Nerve root compression: About 95 percent of the disk prolapse takes place through the L_{4-5} region compressing the L_5 nerve root (Fig. 4.9). The other nerve roots commonly involved are L_4 and S_1 due to disk prolapse between L_{3-4} and L_5–S_1 respectively.

Remember one question test: Radicular pain

Between the knee and the ankle, where is the pain?

- Front →L_4
- Side →L_5
- Back →S_1

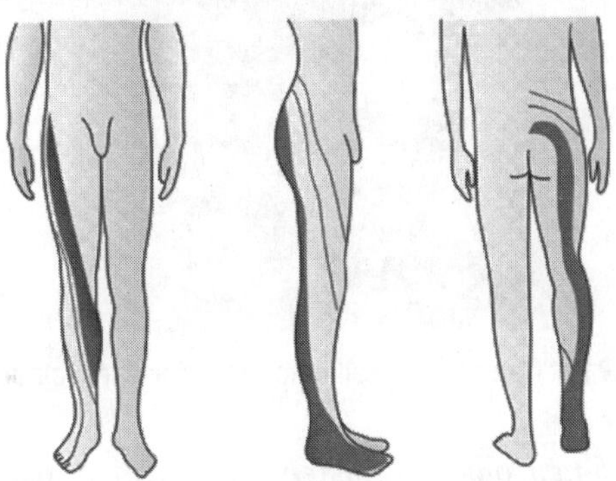

Fig. 4.9: Dermatome pattern from above downwards belong to L_4 L_5 S_1 nerve roots respectively

Examination of the Back

Inspection: Note any postural defects like scoliosis, lordosis or kyphosis. In IVDP there will be loss of lumbar lordosis and the back appears flat (Fig. 4.10).

Palpation consists of:

a. *Tenderness:* Look for the following points:
   - Diffuse tenderness over the lower back
   - Localized tender infiltrates of the skin and subcutaneous tissue.
   - Palpable tender indurations of small intervertebral muscles.
   - Tenderness at the level of posterior articulation of the involved segment and pain on percussion of affected intervertebral space.

b. *Movements:* All the movements of the spine are tested and found to be restricted in all directions.

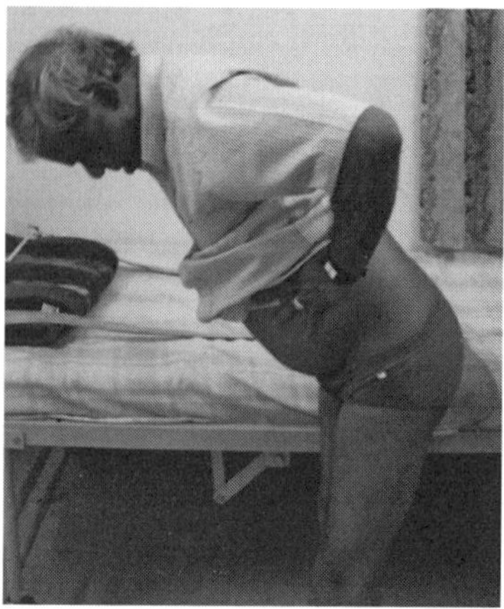

Fig. 4.10: IVDP flat back and inability to bend forward (clinical photo) toes

Evaluation of neurological system: The dermatomal and the myotomal distribution are carefully analyzed to detect the level of lesion.

Clinical tests: These tests are based on the stretching of sciatic nerve over the prolapsed disk:

a. Forward bending to touch the toes.
b. Sitting and alternatively extending one leg and then the other.
c. *Slump test* sitting bent forward and extending one leg and then the other.
d. *Straight leg raising test (SLRT):* Patient is in supine position, the examiner raises the leg straight one after the other. Up to 30°, nerve is not put under stretch. Between 30 and 70°, nerve encounters the prolapsed disk and the patient complains of pain. Beyond 70° if the patient complains of pain, it is usually not due to disk prolapse but could be due to sacroiliac joint involvement.

Modifications of SLRT

- ***Lasègue's test:*** Here, the hip is flexed, knee is flexed and the leg is slowly straightened.

- ***Bückling's sign:*** Perform an SLRT until the patient complains of pain. Now ask the patient to flex the knee. Pain decreases due to relief of tension on the nerve.
- ***Sicard's test:*** After doing SLRT, dorsiflex the great toe. This puts further tension on the sciatic nerve and the patient complains of pain.
- ***Fajersztajn's test:*** After doing SLRT, dorsiflex the foot. This tenses the sciatic nerve and the patient complains of pain.

e. *Well leg raising test:* Here, the patient is asked to perform SLRT of the normal limb. If the patient complains of pain on the affected side, then it is highly suggestive of disk prolapse and this is a pathognomonic test, which has more relevance than the conventional SLRT.

f. *Bilateral straight leg raising test:* Here, patient is asked to raise both the legs simultaneously. This is a test for the sacroiliac joint rather than the spine. During the first 70°, stress is on the SI joint, over 70° stress is on the lumbar spine.

g. *Femoral nerve stretch test (reverse SLRT):* Here, the patient is in prone position and is asked to lift the leg straight. This puts a stretch on the femoral nerve. If the patient complains of pain, it indicates a high level disk prolapse ($L_{1\text{-}2\text{-}3}$).

Remember

About SLRT

- SLRT exerts tension on the sciatic nerve as it passes over the prolapsed disk.
- In disk prolapse SLRT is positive usually between 30° and 70°.
- Many modifications of SLRT either exert more tension (Fajersztajn's test) or relieve tension on the sciatic nerve (Buckling sign).
- Contralateral well leg raising test is more pathognomonic of disk prolapse than SLRT.
- Bilateral leg raising test has more relevance for SI joint pathology than back.
- Reverse leg raising test or femoral nerve stretch test is for detecting high lesion like L_1 root involvement.

Clinical Facts

Diagnosis of the disk disease is a suspect, if:

- Leg pain is minimal and back pain is predominant.
- If pain is bizarre or continuous.
- If the forward bending of the spine is normal.
- If the lumbar spine deviates to the opposite side.
- If tenderness is elicited over the midline.
- *Remember the hallmark of disk disease is repetitive low backache and buttock pain, which is relieved by rest.*
- It is important to note that paresthesiae and motor signs are seen in 96 percent of cases of disk prolapse. Sensory signs are seen in 80 percent. They are distributed along the involved nerve roots as explained earlier.

Remember

Diagnostic clues to detect high level disk lesion involving L_1 and L_2 nerve roots

- Pain in the groin or testicles
- Cauda equina lesion
- Positive femoral stretch test
- Atrophy of the involved limb
- 95 percent of the disk ruptures usually occur at L_4 L_5

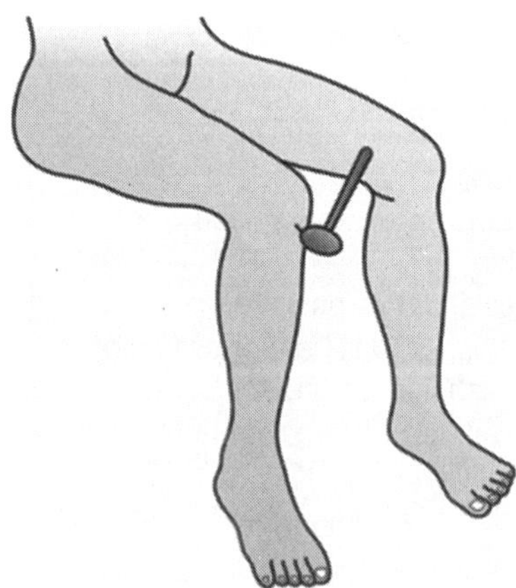

Fig. 4.11: Involvement of L4 myotome (Patient is unable to extend the knee and loss of knee reflex)

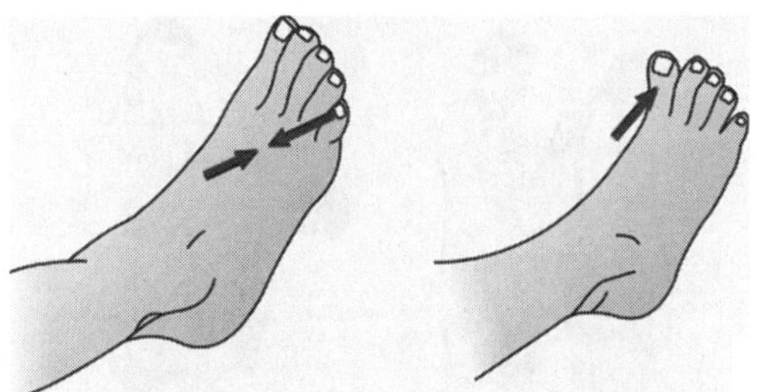

Fig. 4.12: Involvement of L_5 myotome, patient is unable to extend the toes

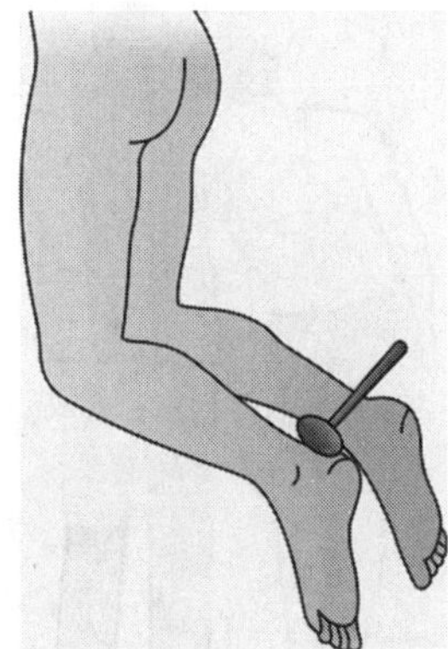

Fig. 4.13: S1 myotome involvement loss of ankle jerk and plantar flexion

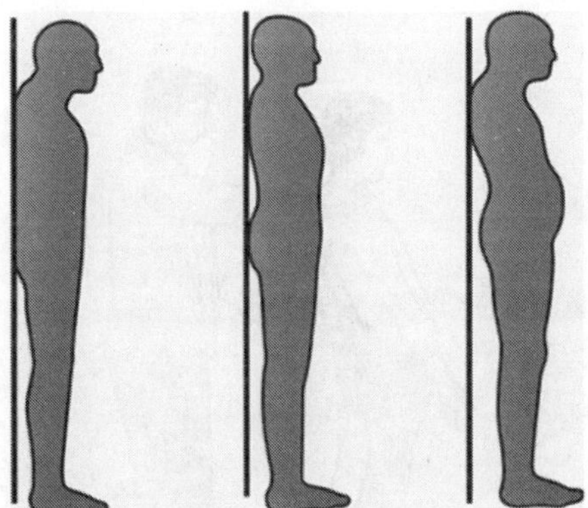

Fig 4.14: Examination of the spine deformities

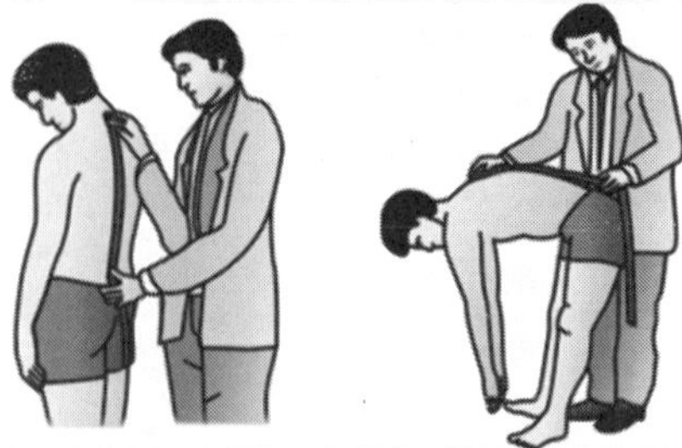

Fig 4.15: Examination of forward flexion

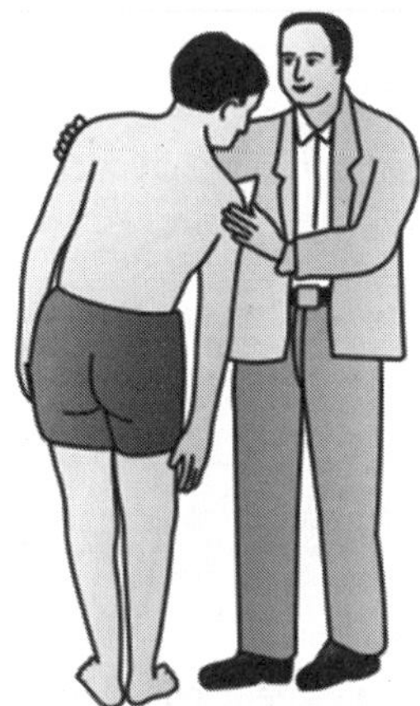

Fig 4.16: Examination of lateral flexion

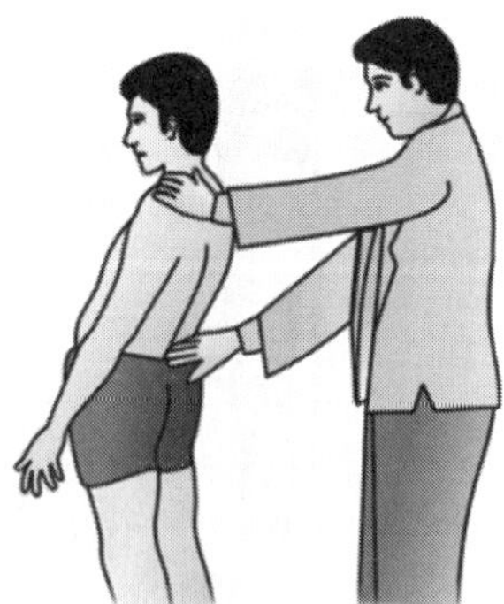

Fig 4.17: Examination of extension

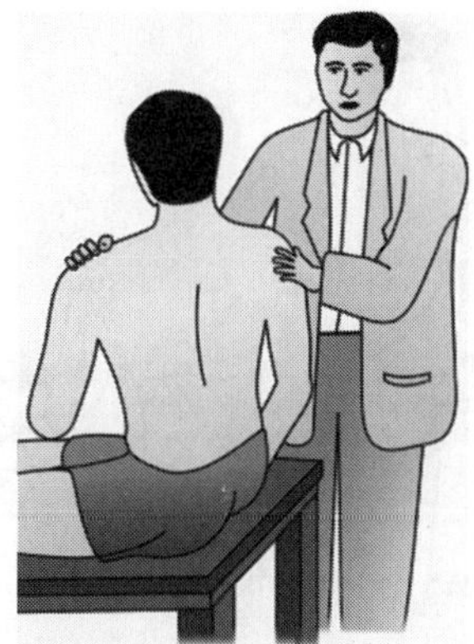

Fig 4.18: Examination of lateral rotation

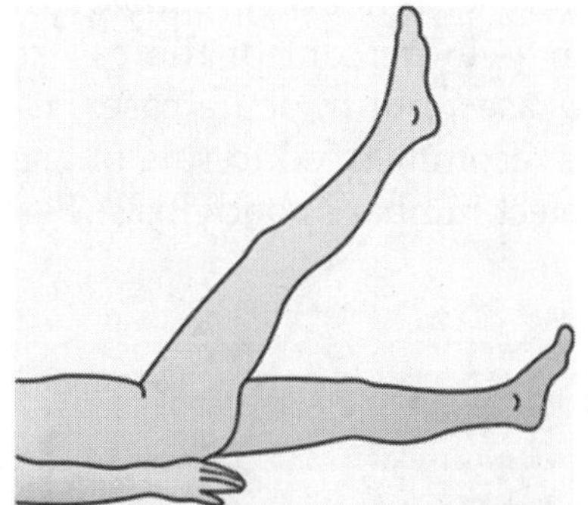

Fig 4.19: Examination of straight leg raising

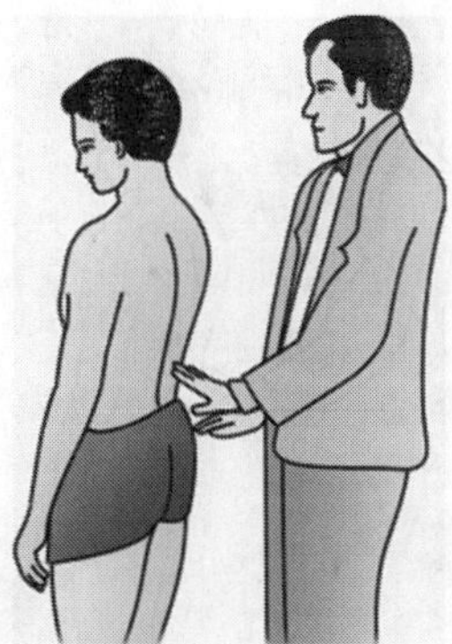

Fig 4.20: Method of eliciting tenderness

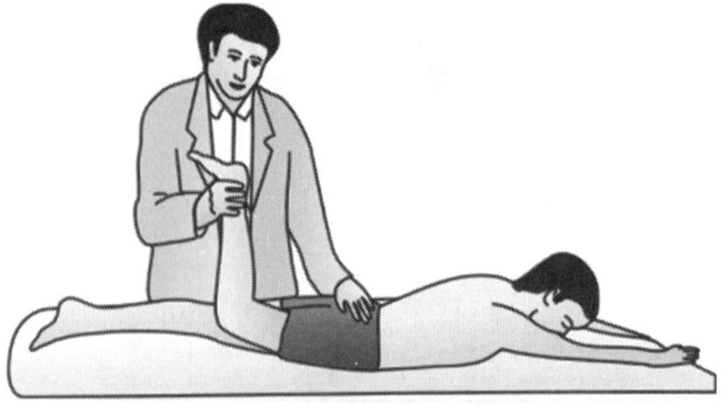

Fig 4.21: Examination of reverse SLRT

Investigations of Low Backache

Radiography of the back is not very reliable as normal findings are observed in 7–46 percent of the cases. Disk space is reduced in old cases; but in acute cases, it is maintained. Oblique view is recommended to rule out spondylolysis. It also helps to detect lumbar spondylosis (Fig. 4.22).

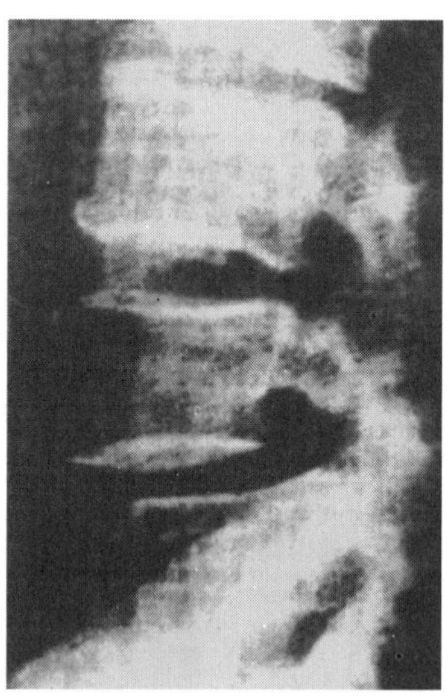

Fig. 4.22: Radiograph showing lumbar spondylosis

Myelography consists of injecting radiopaque dye (Myodil was used earlier now it is the water-soluble Iopamiro 300, which is being used) into the spinal canal and taking radiographs of the back. It is helpful in detecting the intraspinal lesions, spinal stenosis and cases of previously operated (Fig. 4.23) backs. It is also indicated when the diagnosis is in doubt. It is an invasive procedure and is no longer performed. It is now replaced by noninvasive procedures like CT scan and MRI.

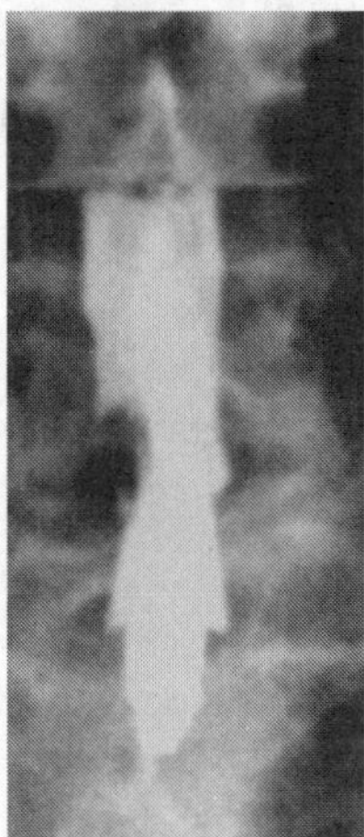

Fig. 4.23: Myelographic study of the lumbar spine

CT scan: It is a very useful noninvasive, painless outpatient procedure. It gives a crosssectional study of the pathology. It, however, fails to detect intra-spinal lesion, arachnoiditis and scar from disk herniation. It helps to detect the foraminal stenosis and the lateral disk prolapse (Fig. 4.24).

MRI: This is also an extremely useful, painless, non-invasive outpatient procedure. It helps to detect the intraspinal lesion, helps to examine the entire spine and identifies degenerative disk (Figs 4.25). However, it is expensive and hence prohibitive.

Discography: After identifying the disk correctly, through a needle, a radiopaque dye is injected into the space. This reproduces the pain experienced by the patient previously and is relieved by injecting Xylocaine. This confirms the diagnosis. It is a painful procedure and can introduce infection into the disk. Hence, it is less practiced.

Other tests of diagnostic importance are *bone scans, EMG,* routine laboratory studies, injection studies, etc.

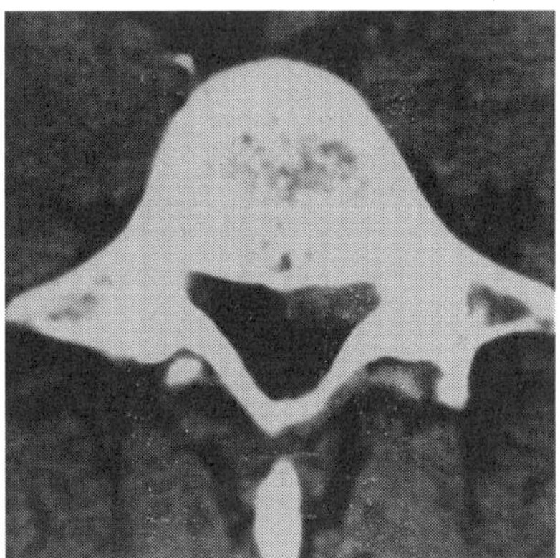

Fig. 4.24: CT scan showing posterolateral disc herniation

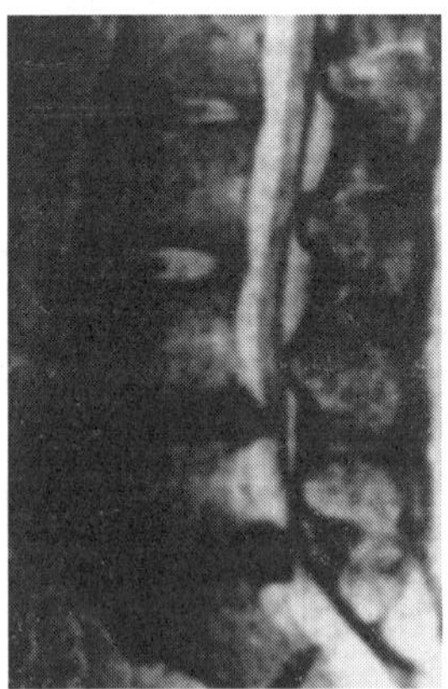

Fig. 4.25: MRI of lumbar spine showing bilateral disc prolapse

Differential Diagnosis

There are many causes for lower backache. The most common one being lumbar disk disease due to abnormal posture and aging process. The differential diagnosis is as follows:

Extrinsic Causes (unrelated to spine)

Diseases of the:
- Urogenital system
- Gastrointestinal system
- Vascular system
- Endocrine system
- Nervous system
- Musculoskeletal system, etc.

Intrinsic Causes (related to spine)

Important Causes
- Unstable spondylolisthesis
- Osteoporosis and compression of the vertebrae
- Marked loss of disk height at multiple levels
- Severe scoliosis.

Unimportant Causes
- Lumbar spondylosis
- Mild discopathy
- Arthroses of the facet joints
- Disk calcification
- Spina bifida
- Schmorl's nodes
- Mild-to-moderate scoliosis.

Predominant cause of backache as already suggested is lumbar disk disease. Common diseases that mimic lumbar disk disease include ankylosing spondylitis, multiple myeloma, vascular insufficiency, arthritis of the hip joint, osteoporosis with stress fractures, extradural tumors, peripheral neuropathy, herpes zoster, etc.

Do you know the common diagnosis of low backache?

Well, here is a list:

- Common low backache (disk disease, muscle and ligament strain and sprain of the back)
- Myofascial pain
- Spondylosis
- Spondylolisthesis
- Facet syndrome
- Fibromyalgia
- Lumbar canal stenosis

Pitfalls: Only in 15 percent of the cases of low backaches, accurate diagnosis of a specific cause can be made.

Treatment of Low Backache due to Lumbar Disk Disease

Principles of Treatment

The principles of treating low backache due to lumbar disk disease are explained by **three Rs**:

- **R**elieve pain in acute cases.
- **R**estore normal movements in chronic cases.
- **R**ecurrence is to be prevented.

The following are the treatment modalities in low backache.

Conservative therapy: *Absolute bed rest is the best treatment for acute low backache.* Ice packs, nonsteroidal anti-inflammatory drugs (NSAIDs), muscle relaxants, anti-depressants are recommended. Bucks extension skin traction and pelvic traction helps to relieve pain. Walking within limits of comfort is also encouraged. Sitting and riding in a car is discouraged. Back braces or belts are recommended in acute stages. They are discarded as soon as symptoms decrease; otherwise, muscles become weak and hasten the degeneration.

Role of exercises: As the pain decreases, isometric abdominal and lower extremity exercises are begun. Choice of exercises is based on the increase or decrease of pain by extension or flexion. *If pain decreases by extension, extension exercises are recommended. On the other hand, if the pain decreases by flexion, flexion exercises are recommended. Improvements in symptoms with extension are indication of a good prognosis with conservative care.* Lower extremity exercises increase the strength and relieve the stress on the back, but they may increase the lower extremity arthritis. Thus, the true benefit of such treatment may be in the promotion of good posture and body mechanics than strength.

Back education and importance of proper posture is taught.

See the pictorial display of proper postural habits and back exercises recommended for prevention of low backache (Figs 4.26 to 4.31).

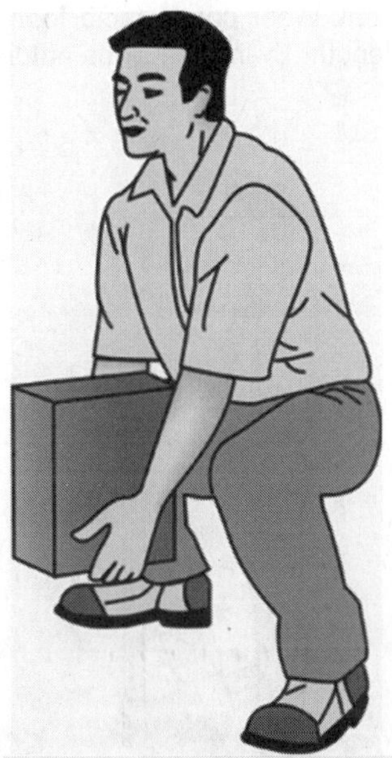

Fig. 4.26: Lifting objects: Bend at your knees and not at your waist. Hold the object you are lifting close to your body, not higher than your chest. It is easier to push rather than pull heavy objects, e.g. furniture, and keep the knees bent while pushing

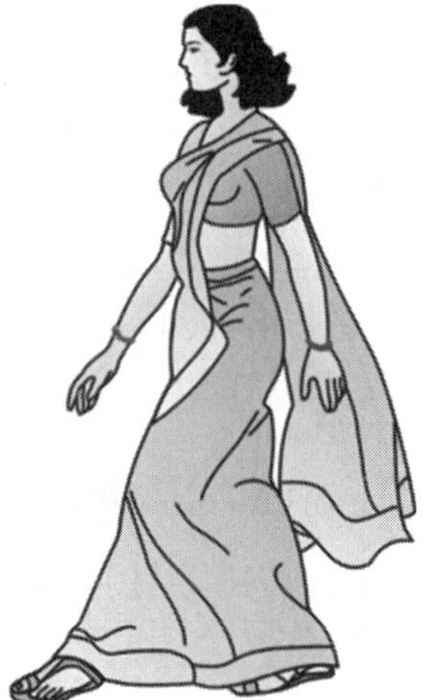

Fig. 4.27: Walking: Walk well with your head high, chin tucked in, toes pointing straight in front. Wear comfortable footwear. Take steps of a natural, comfortable length. Swing the arms naturally

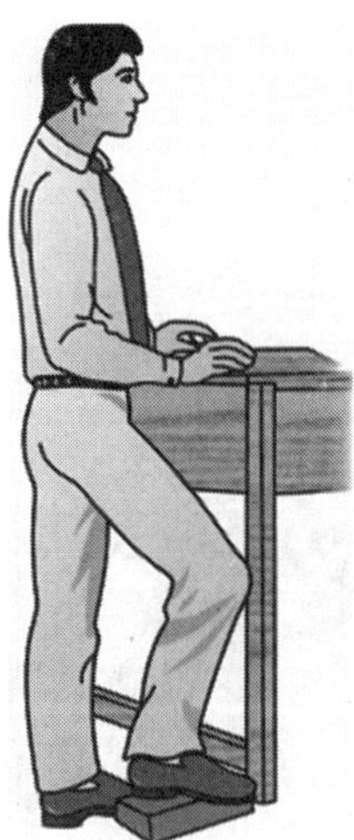

Fig. 4.28: Standing: Keep one foot in front and knees slightly bent while standing upright. If you have to stand for a long time, try keeping one foot higher than the other does, on a low stool. Change your position often

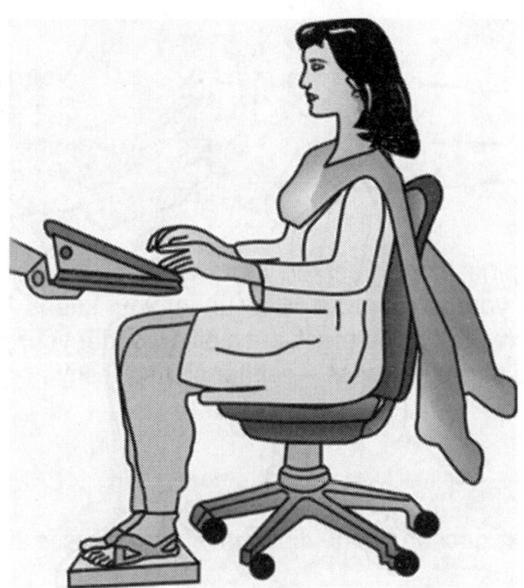

Fig. 4.29: Sitting: Ensure your back is firmly touching the back of the chair. Keep the knees slightly higher than the hips, e.g. by using something to prop up your feet. Sit close to your desk or table to avoid bending forward. Do not sit for too long. In addition, when driving, move the front seat close to the steering wheel and both hands should be kept on the wheel

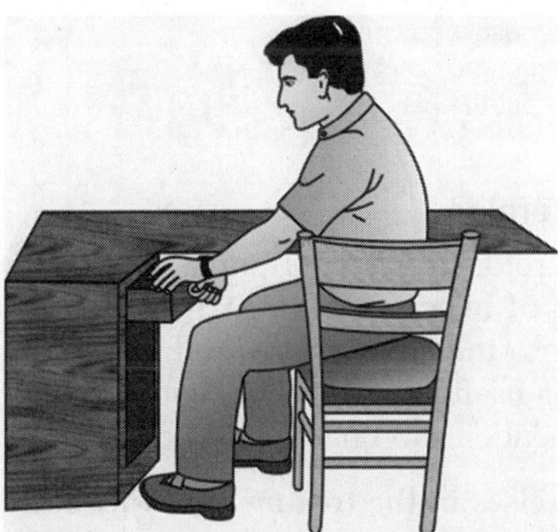

Fig. 4.30: Turning and reaching out: Do not twist your waist. Rather, turn by moving your feet. Keep the phone and such like objects within easy reach; do not strain to reach them. Stand on a stool to reach high objects

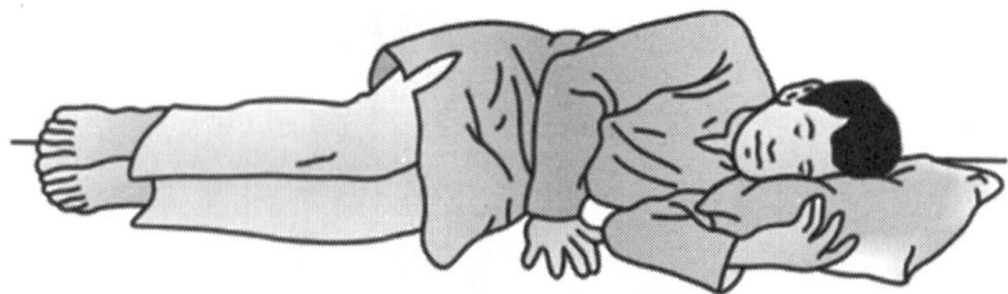

Fig. 4.31: Sleeping: If you sleep on your side, keep knees and lower body bent a little. On your back, put a pillow under your knees. Try not to sleep on your stomach—but if you must, put a pillow under your waist not under your head. Use a firm mattress—neither soft/squashy nor very hard

Did you know?

Maximal load reduction on the disk with tight corsets is 20–30 percent.

Remember

Contraindications to traction

- Hypertension
- Peripheral vascular disease
- Cataracts and glaucoma
- Labile asthma or COPD
- Pregnancy, etc.

How traction helps?

- It relieves muscle spasm
- It may distract the facet joints
- It may distract the disk space

Epidural Steroids

Epidural steroids are a symptomatic method of treatment, and consist of injecting a longacting steroid and a local anesthetic into the epidural space. Its effect lasts for three weeks and is useful for sub acute and chronic cases. It also reduces dependence on narcotics in chronic cases.

Role of exercises in the treatment of low backache

Back stretching and strengthening exercises are an important form of treatment for the low backache. It plays a very important role both in the prevention and cure of backache.

All about epidural steroid injection

- In vogue since 1950s.
- Effective in approximately 50 percent patients with low backache.
- It decreases inflammation and flushes out inflammatory proteins thereby reducing pain.
- It helps in better back rehabilitation.
- Maximum of three injections in a year with a two-week gap is given.
- Adverse features include infection, dural puncture and arachnoiditis.
- It primarily decreases leg pain.
- After the injection, the patient is advised one-day rest.

See the pictorial display of proper back exercises recommended for prevention of low backache (Figs 4.32 to 4.37).

How does exercise relieve low backache?

- Exercises pump the disk and increase water content.
- Relieves the muscle spasm and increase motion.
- Stretches and mobilizes the facet joints.
- Repetitive motion helps the patient to overcome the fear of movement.
- Decreases the swelling around the nerves.

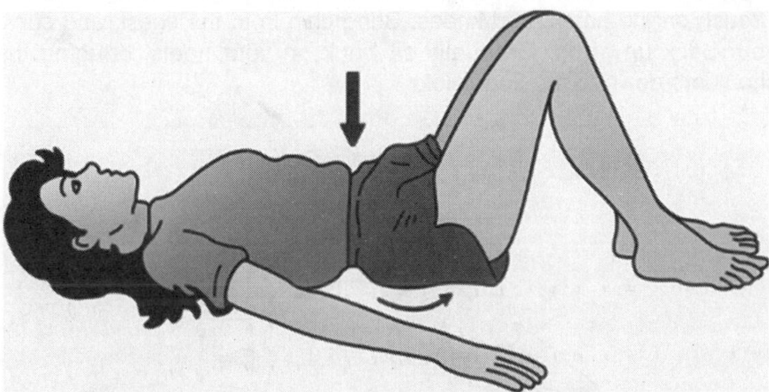

Fig. 4.32: Pelvic tilt: Makes abdominal muscles stronger. Lie on your back, legs bent, and feet flat on the floor with arms to your sides. Push your lower back against the floor—your hips will tilt up. Hold this position for a short while

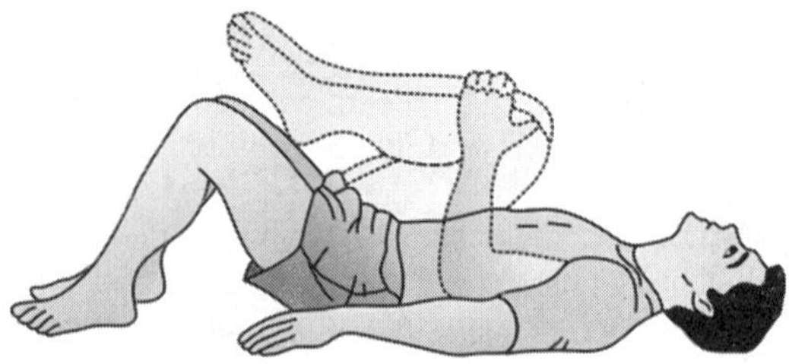

Fig. 4.33: Knees to chest: Lie on your back, knees bent, feet flat, and arms to your sides. Raise first one knee to your chest, then the other, holding them with your hands as shown (or just inside your knee). Bring legs down one at a time and rest. Repeat

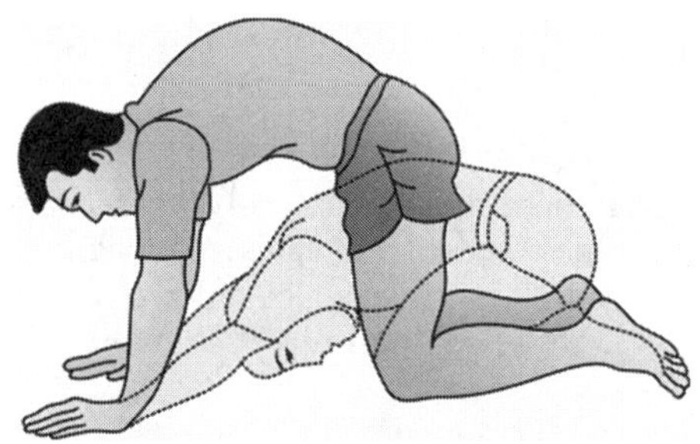

Fig. 4.34: Trunk flex: Stretches the back, abdominal and leg muscles. Crouch on the hands and knees. Bring chin in to the chest, and curve your back upwards. Gradually sit back on your heels, bringing the shoulders down to the floor. Hold

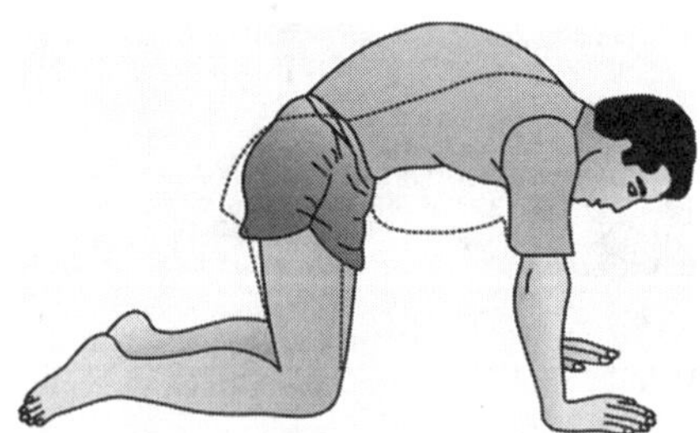

Fig. 4.35: Cat and Camel: Strengthens the back and abdominal muscles. Crouch on hands and knees. Keeping the head parallel to floor, arch your back and then let it gradually sag towards the floor by breathing out. Keep the arms straight

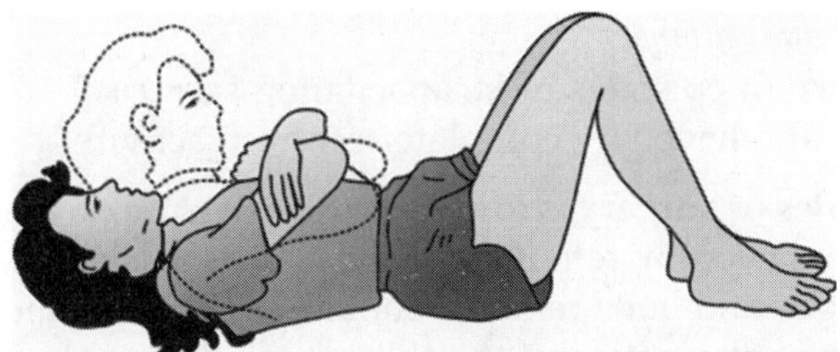

Fig. 4.36: Semi sit-up: Strengthens the abdominal muscles. Lie with your back and feet flat on the floor, knees bent, arms folded on the chest. Lift only your head and shoulders off the floor and hold. Repeat, trying to hold longer each time

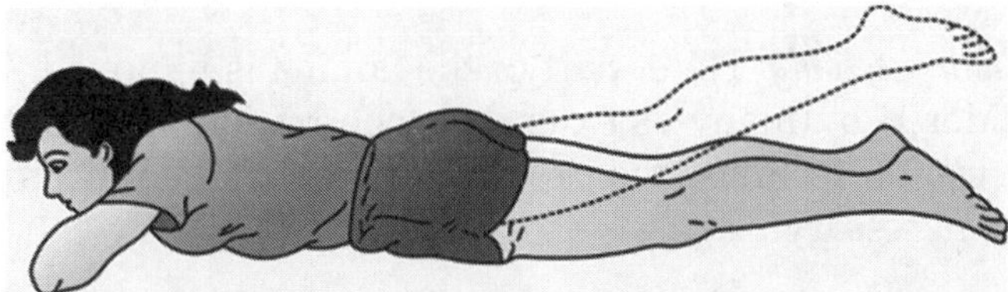

Fig. 4.37: Hip stretch: Strengthens and stretches hip, buttock and back muscles. Lie on the stomach, arms folded under the chin. Slowly lift one leg without bending, but not too high. Lower it and raise the other leg. Keep pelvis in contact with the floor

Note:
- Each exercise is done one to five times twice daily.
- The number of repetitions should be kept increasing to reach a minimum of ten repetitions twice daily.
- Exercises are to be done slowly and smoothly.

Surgery

What are the indications for surgery?

Absolute indications

- Failed conservative management.
- Marked progressive weakness of muscles.
- Progressive neurological deficit.
- Cauda equina paralysis.

Relative indications

- Recurrent episodes of incapacitating sciatica.
- Pain unrelieved by complete rest from activity.

Principles of surgery is to see that the pressure on the nerve root is relieved by removing the prolapsed disk. Dissection of muscles and bone removal should be kept at a minimum to prevent weakening of the spine.

Surgical Methods

Laminectomy and disk excision earlier, this was the surgery of choice; but now, it is no longer resorted to as it makes the spine unstable.

Hemilaminectomy: Here, part of the lamina is removed. It is considered by many as extended fenestration approach. If fenestration technique is properly done, hemilaminectomy is not necessary.

Fenestration surgery here, the spine is approached unilaterally and the spine on the opposite side is not exposed. Here, only the contiguous margin of upper and lower laminae is removed and medial facetectomy is done. The disk is now excised. This procedure requires that MRI and radiographic studies correctly locate the affected disk.

Microscopic and endoscopic lumbar discectomy (Fig. 4.38): Using an operating microscope or an endoscope, the disk can be excised through a very small incision (< 3.5 cm) with minimum damage to the structures and minimal blood loss. It is a technically demanding procedure and gives excellent results if done in properly indicated cases like a single level posterolateral disk prolapse. The patient can be discharged home within two days and he or she can return to his or her normal work faster. In short, it can be described as a less invasive, less painful, more specific procedure giving maximum comforts to the patient. *Dr PS Ramani calls it as "come today, go tomorrow" surgery!*

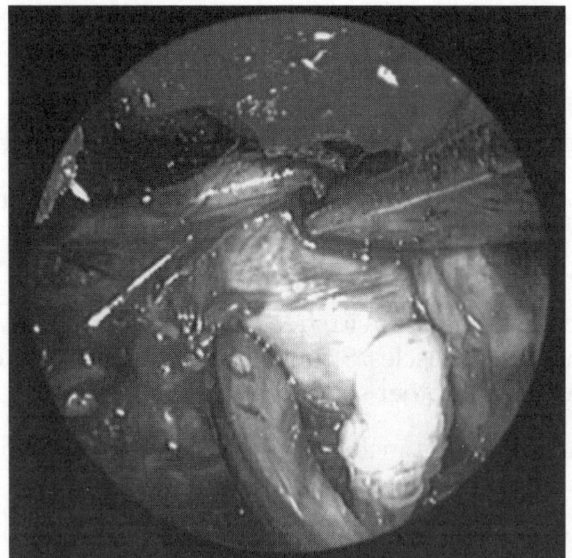

Fig. 4.38: Microscopic lumbar discectomy (MLD)

What is new in the treatment of low backache?

- MISS (Minimally invasive spinal surgery) this consists of endoscopic spine surgery discectomy and was popularized by John Chiu.
- Laser diskectomy
- Percutaneous discectomy (manual or automated)
- *Total disk replacement (TDR):* Total or partial disk replacement using a prosthetic disk nucleus for IVDP. It has a hydrogel core and is encased in a polyethylene jacket. It restores disk height and ensures normal range of mobility.

Chemonucleolysis

Indications are the same as for surgery. It is limited to lumbar spine. Drug used is chymopapain.

Ways to Prevent Recurrence

This is the most important aspect of the management of backache. *Like in all other diseases, so in backache prevention is better than cure. Backache can be prevented largely by observing the following measures:*

Adopting proper posture and creating awareness that it is in the erect position that the back can withstand strain the best.

Back education: Stress on the back is less when it is properly used during sitting, walking, etc. These proper habits have to be cultivated with practice.

Back exercises: These aim to strengthen the abdominal, pelvic, back and thigh muscles. Strong healthy muscles reduce load on the disks and other structures.

To avoid: All sports including the aerobic ones. Swimming and walking are encouraged.

Treatment plan of backache due to disk disease

Conservative	• Absolute bed rest • Traction • NSAIDs • Belts
Epidural steroids	• For sub acute and chronic cases • Long-acting steroids + Local anesthetics • Reduces dependence on narcotics • Effect lasts for 3 weeks
Surgery	• Done in proper indications • Open or microscopic or endoscopic lumbar discectomy
Chemonucleolysis	• Same indications as for surgery • Limited only to lumbar spine • Drug used is chymopapain
Physiotherapy	• Active and passive physiotherapy • Flexion or extension exercises
Recurrence prevention	• Back education • Proper postural habits • Back exercises • Avoid all sports

Remember

Consider serious causes of backache if any one of the following situations is encountered

- Pain in patients less than 10 years of age
- First time backache in patients greater than 60 years
- Unexplained weight loss
- Chronic cough
- Night pains
- Intermenstrual bleeding
- Altered bowel function
- Altered bladder control
- Visual disturbances and balance problems.

Remember the Do's and Don'ts

Do's

- Forward bent attitude.
- Body weight borne on the heels.
- Proper weightlifting as shown earlier.
- Sit with buttocks tucked under.
- While driving, push the seat forwards to raise the knees and decrease the lordosis.
- Flex the knees and hip when lying on the side.
- Turn to the side and then get up.

Don'ts

- Sleep in the prone position.
- Rise from a sitting position suddenly.
- Bend over a washbasin.
- Wear high heels as pelvis is thrust forward and the spine bends backward.
- Use too high a chair.
- Use soft mattress, which increases the lumbosacral extension. A firm mattress encourages lumbar spine to be straight.

Remember Bs in backache

- **B**ad posture
- **B**ed rest
- **B**elts
- **B**ack education
- **B**ack exercises
- **B**ed choice

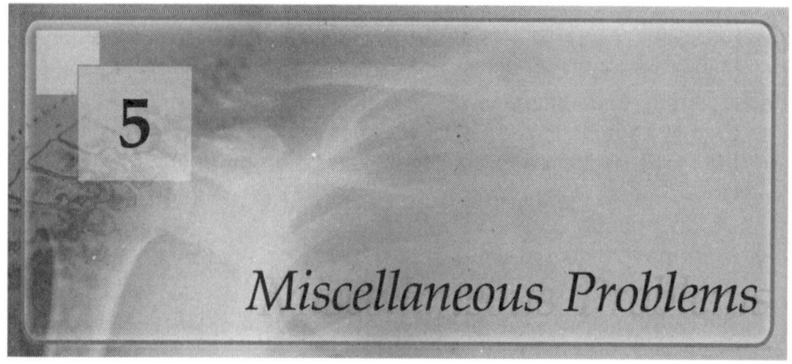

REPETITIVE STRESS INJURIES
(Also called Computer Related Injuries)

Introduction

This is a new epidemic seen across the globe. Computers have no doubt revolutionized our lives in many ways, so much so that it is hard to imagine our lives without them. But it has its darker sides too. ***Working extensively on computers in a improper way for a long time*** can cause an overuse injury affecting the soft tissues like the muscles, tendons, ligaments, nerves of the neck, shoulder, upper and lower back, arms and hands.

Who is at risk?

This is a moot point. Generally any one who uses computers for more than one hour per day are at risk and this includes the following groups:

- Software professionals.
- Bank employees.
- Call centre workers.
- Children and elderly.
- Musicians, Barbers, Butchers.
- Clerks, Stenotypists, Assembly line workers.

Incidence: About 15–25% of computer users across the glove are at risk of developing this problem. About 75% of the IT

Professionals are affected with RSI at some stage of their career.

RSI IS A WORK RELATED MUSCULOSKELETAL INJURIES (MSIs)

RSI is a work related musculoskeletal injuries (MSIs) affecting the upper body, neck, back and lower limbs and are now recognized as one of the leading causes of worker pain and disability. A work-related musculoskeletal disorder is an injury to the muscles, tendons and/or nerves of the upper body either caused or aggravated by work. Other names used to describe work-related musculoskeletal disorders include repetitive motion injuries, repetitive strain injuries, cumulative trauma disorders, soft tissue disorders and overuse syndromes.

Musculoskeletal disorders, including carpal tunnel syndrome, are among the most prevalent medical conditions in the US, affecting 7% of the population. They account for 14% of physician visits and 19% of hospital stays. 62% of the persons with musculoskeletal disorders report some degree of limitation on activity, compared with 14% of the population at large, according to the National Institute for Occupational Safety and Health.

Musculoskeletal disorders are the country's most costly category of workplace injuries and illnesses. In addition to spending $20 billion annually on workers' compensation costs due to RSIs, the US spends another $100 billion on lost productivity, employee turnover, and other indirect expenses; The Agency for Health Care Policy and Research.

Causes of RSI

- Poor Posture
- Repetitive Motion
- Trauma
- Lifestyle without ergonomic care, e.g. While working in front of computers, driving, traveling.

- Simple reasons like 'Using a blunt knife for everyday chopping of vegetables', may cause RSI.
- Reading or doing tasks for extended periods of time while looking down.
- Sleeping on an inadequate bed/mattress or sitting in a bad armchair and/or in an uncomfortable position.
- Carrying heavy items.
- Holding one's phone between neck and shoulder.
- Watching TV in incorrect position, e.g. Too much to the left/right.
- Sleeping with head forward, while traveling.
- Prolonged use of the hands, wrists, back, neck, etc.

Presentation: RSI can affect one or more of the following structures:

Neck: It can cause acute and chronic neck pains. In the long run it may predispose to cervical spondylosis.

Eyes: It may affect the vision and cause irritation and blurring.

Shoulder: Shoulder pain is a very common complaint.

Elbow: It can lead to Tennis elbow, Golfers elbow, pain within the wrist joint, etc.

Forearm: Forearm muscle cramps, fatigue, etc.

Wrist: It can lead to carpal tunnel syndrome, wrist pain, etc.

Fingers: It can cause pain in the fingers. There could be a feeling of tingling and numbness of the fingers.

Backache: This is a frequent complaint and can affect the upper, middle or lower back.

So looking at the long list of complaints makes one weary of this problem and calls for effective preventive and curative measures to tackle this ugly menace.

Symptoms

- Symptoms of repetitive stress injury may occur anywhere in the shoulders or arms.

- Usually they first occur during the repetitive movement.
- These first symptoms may include tired muscles, aches, and pain.

Later, if repetitive movement continues, the symptoms worsen and may include:

- Muscles aches
- Muscle fatigue, During activity and at rest
- Tingling sensation in the affected area
- Pain radiating up the arm
- Difficulty in sleeping
- Numbness in the affected area, Especially the fingers
- Disability because of chronic pain or weakness
- Frustration and depression due to pain

The following complaints are typical in patients of RSI:

- Short bursts of excruciating pain in the arm, back, shoulders, wrists, hands, or thumbs (typically diffuse – i.e. spread over many areas).
- The pain is worse with activity.
- Weakness, lack of endurance.

The physical examination discloses only

- Tenderness and
- Diminished performance on effort-based tests such as grip and pinch strength
- No other objective abnormalities are present.
- Diagnostic tests (*radiological, electrophysiological, etc.*) are normal.

> *Note:* In short, RSI is best understood as an apparently healthy arm that hurts. Whether there is currently undetectable damage remains to be established.

The symptoms hallmark of RSI mtend to be

- Diffuse and non-anatomical,
- Crossing the distribution of nerves, tendons, etc.
- They tend not to be characteristic of any discrete pathological conditions.

Why does RSI happen in the computer professionals?

A look at the list provides the answer:

- Improper use of the computers.
- The mouse and the keyboard placed at uncomfortable heights and positions.
- Very hard keyboards or forceful typing over them.
- Height of the monitors kept at uncomfortable levels.

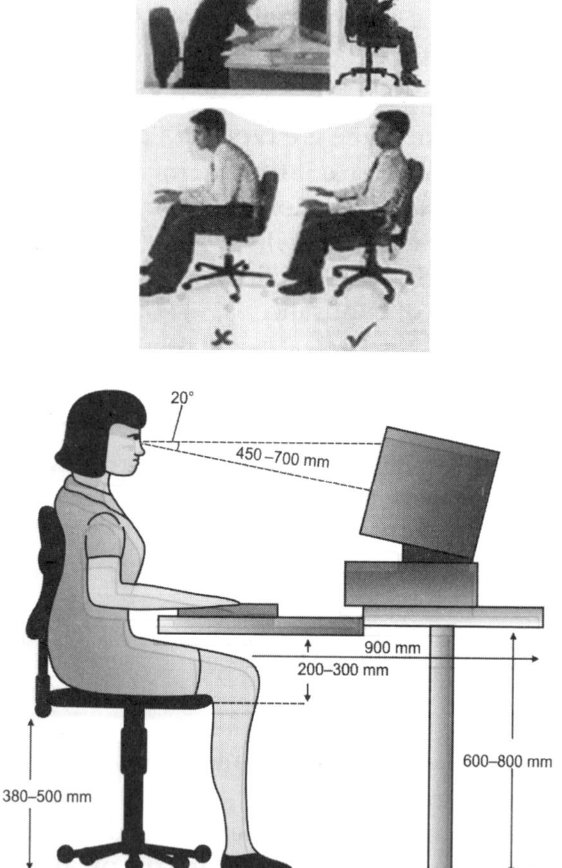

Fig. 5.1: Causes for RSI (above) and the remedy (below)

- Improper postures of the neck and back while working.
- Poorly designed unscientific working chairs.
- Extreme mental and physical stress.

Stages: This disease runs through the following stages:

First stage: Here symptoms are seen only at work.

Second stage: Here symptoms persist but disappear with rest.

Third stage: Here the symptoms are permanent.

Types of RSI

RSI are divided into two main categories:

Type 1 RSI

This includes well defined syndromes such as

- Carpal tunnel syndrome (pain and compression in the wrist)
- Tendonitis (inflammation of a tendon),
- Tenosynovitis (inflammation of a tendon sheath) etc.
- These conditions may be due to, or be made worse by, repetitive tasks.
- However, these syndromes are also common in people who have not done repetitive tasks.
- These syndromes may have other symptoms such as swelling, inflammation, nerve compression problems, etc.

Type 2 RSI

- Here symptoms do not fit into a well defined syndrome.
- There are no 'objective' or 'measurable' signs such as inflammation, swelling or problems with nerve function.
- It is sometimes called 'diffuse RSI' or 'non-specific pain syndrome'.

Diagnosis and Tests

The diagnosis of repetitive stress injury begins with a complete medical history and physical examination. The doctor may order tests like:

- X-Rays and other imaging scans, Such as an MRI
- A nerve conduction velocity test (NCV) to check for nerve damage.
- Blood tests, Including a complete blood count (CBC), to rule out infection.
- A biopsy of any fluid or growths to rule out infection, tumor, or cancer.

Remedies: In this condition too, prevention is better than cure. The recommended preventive and awareness measures are:
- Awareness about this problem.
- Proper postures during work.
- Using ergonomically designed chairs.
- The neck, elbow and shoulder should be placed at a comfortable height.
- The height of the computer monitor should be just above the eye level
- Taking breaks from typing at every five minutes, fifteen and half an hour of typing.
- Taking a short break after every half an hour. Getting up, taking a short walk and sitting against for work is a good practice.
- Neck, shoulder, back, elbow and fingers stretchs help to relive pain and stress.
- Yoga and meditation helps to combat mental and physical stress.
- Keeping realistic goals and philosophical attitude defuses mental tension and prevents burn out.

Curative Measures: Treatment of problems like neck pain, shoulder pain, elbow problems like tennis elbow, wrist problems like compartment syndrome have been dealt in relevant books. (I suggest you to read my book on Shoulder, Pain and Wrist conditions). However, in the event of pain your doctor suggests the following general measures:
- *Drugs:* Pain killers like NSAIDs are the drugs of choice. The more popular ones belong to nimesulides, rofecoxib,

valedocoxib, diclofenac sodium, etc. They are preferably taken for short spells and that too after consultation and recommendation from hour doctor.

- *Physiotherapy:* This consists of gentle massage, heat therapies like hot water packs, TENS, Ultrasound, Short wave diathermy, etc.
- *Exercises:* Once the pain subsides, patient is instructed to carry out suitable neck, shoulder, elbow and finger exercises.
- *Surgery:* This is rarely required.

Health education: This is the most important aspect of tackling this highly preventable problem. The aspects mentioned in the above columns have to be scrupulously enforced to keep this problem at bay.

Ergonomics (Role of the insititutions): Institutions should provide good working conditions and facilities to all its workers. Good illumination, recreation facilities, and realistic workloads go a long way in helping the employees cope with

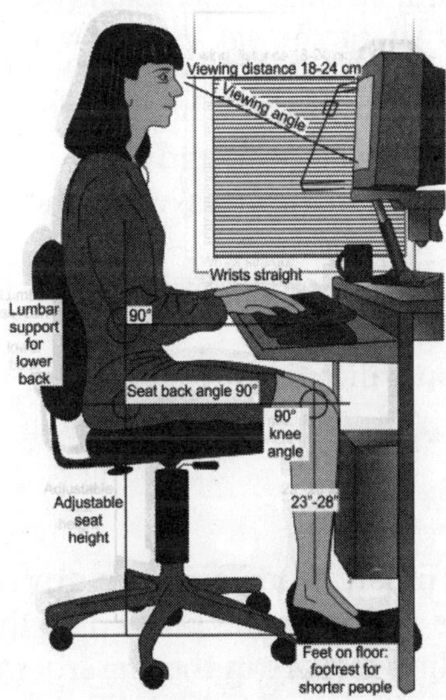

Fig. 5.2: Recommended specification for working on a computer

this problem. Modifications of posture and arm use (*ergonomics*) are often recommended.

Ergonomics: The science of designing the job, equipment, and workplace.

BACKACHE IN SPECIAL SITUATIONS

BACKACHE IN CHILDREN (School Bag Syndrome)

It is indeed very pathetic that backache is no longer an unknown entity in children. Thanks to the practice of heavy school bags, the tender backs of children are subjected to untold misery.

Vital facts

Ideally, a child should not carry a bag of >10 percent of his or her body weight. Nevertheless, the scenario in present-day children's life is very different.

Features

We can call this school bag related problems in a child as "school bag stress syndrome". Its features are:

- Pain in the shoulders, neck and back
- Tingling sensation in the arms, wrist and hands especially at night.
- Head and neck are tilted to one side (postural imbalance)
- Frequent headaches
- An uncommon gait.

Prevention

Policy Matter

The school administrations and the government should devise strategies to lessen the burden of the books on the children. Providing lockers in the classrooms, reducing the number of books to be carried, giving less homework are some of the options. However, nothing seems to be happening over this front. Hence, the following improvizations can be tried:

- To use ergonomically designed school bags (Orthofix or orthogrip bags) (Fig. 5.3).
- These bags are easy on the shoulder and back.
- They sit against the curve of the back
- They are provided with good padding for the bagstraps, so that it does not burrow the skin (see box for safe school bag instructions).

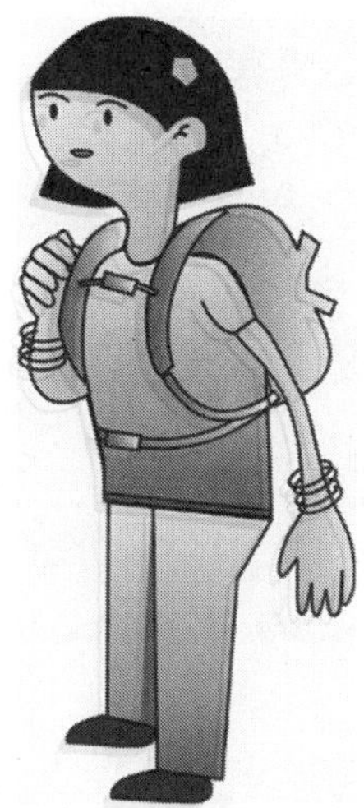

Fig.5.3: Proper school bag carrying technique

Facts vital for school children (Safe School Bag Practice)

- Use an ergonomically designed school bag
- Use both straps to carry the bag
- The knapsack should have several compartments for equal weight distribution
- Heavy items are packed at the top so that weight is borne on the legs instead of the spine
- Both the straps should be worn across the shoulder and upper back to equalize the weight.

Index

Clinical Notes

Clinical Notes